SURGERY

FACTS AND FIGURES

By

James Green LLM, FRCS

Specialist Registrar in Urology
North Thames Deanery

and

Saj Wajed MA, FRCS

Specialist Registrar in Surgery
North Thames Deanery

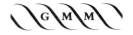

© 2000

GREENWICH MEDICAL MEDIA LTD
137 Euston Road
London
NW1 2AA

ISBN 1 900 151 340

First Published 2000

British Library Cataloguing in Publication Data
A catalogue record for this book is available from the British Library.

Typeset by Saxon Graphics Ltd, Derby

Printed in the UK by the Alden Group, Oxford

Contents

Introduction

USING THIS BOOK

This book has been written to provide relevant information in a condensed and straight-forward manner, through simple paragraphs, tables and diagrams. It attempts to cover the breadth of the present syllabus as notified by the four colleges, and provides the depth of information necessary to attempt the examination. The book is intended to reflect the requirements of the examining boards as closely as possible and will be updated to mirror future changes as and when they arise.

THE EXAMINATION

The examination format has undergone radical change for the MRCS. At present there is a multiple-choice written answer paper, followed by the clinical examination, if sufficient marks have been obtained in the written examination. The change from a written short answer/long answer paper to an MCQ has advantages and disadvantages. While there is no longer the need to formulate a written response, a simple true/false answer must now be given, instead of a discussion of a number of options which was the case previously.

This book will provide the spectrum of questions that may be asked in the exam.

COMMONLY USED ABBREVIATIONS

- Df – definition
- DD – differential diagnosis
- M – male
- F – female
- p.a. – per annum
- 5YS – 5-year survival
- 10YS – 10-year survival
- INR – International Normalized Ratio
- = – equal
- > – greater than
- < less than
- ? – query
- ~ – approximately

METHODS FOR ANSWERING SURGICAL QUESTIONS

Most questions in surgery are related to aetiology, pathology, diagnosis, treatment or prognosis. But if time is tight the most important headings in discussing a disease (in the STEP course) appear to be *definition*, *causes*, *type (grading) clinical features* and *treatment*.

Aetiology

To answer a question on aetiology the 'surgical sieve' can be used:

Congenital

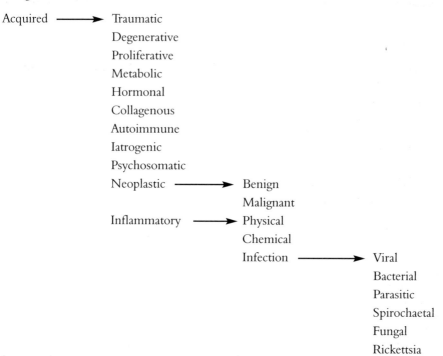

Acquired ⟶ Traumatic
Degenerative
Proliferative
Metabolic
Hormonal
Collagenous
Autoimmune
Iatrogenic
Psychosomatic
Neoplastic ⟶ Benign
Malignant
Inflammatory ⟶ Physical
Chemical
Infection ⟶ Viral
Bacterial
Parasitic
Spirochaetal
Fungal
Rickettsia

Pathology

When discussing pathology the simple mnemonic popularised by Harold Ellis *In A Surgeons Gown a Physician Might Make Some Progress* can be followed:

- Incidence – lung, colorectal, breast, prostate, gastric, etc.
- Age
- Sex
- Geographical
- Predisposing factors
- Macro pathology
- Micro pathology
- Spread/complication (local, general) – in cancer – local, haematogenous, lymphatic, transcoloemic
- Progress or prognosis

Diagnosis

Diagnosis can be broken down into diagnosis of a primary or secondary condition and the general features of malignant or severe disease:

- History (symptoms, acute/chronic)
- Exam (signs)
- General investigations (urine analysis, blood tests)
- Specific investigations (to localize, exclude differentials).

Always start with simple investigations and think of the differential diagnosis and ways to exclude them.

Treatment

In the treatment of cancer and severe disease the following should be taken into account:

- General condition of the patient
- Age and wishes of the patient
- Degree of symptoms
- Severity of the disease (comprises)
  - Stage of disease
    - Local spread – **T**
    - Regional spread – **N**
    - Distal spread – **M**
  - Grade/severity of disease

Management

This can be:

- Preventative
- Prophylactic
- Curative★
- Neoadjuvant
- Adjuvant
- Palliative★★

comprising a choice of modalities : surgery, medical/conservative, chemotherapy, radiotherapy, hormonal, immunosuppressive.

In cancer there are four general types of tumours to manage:

Tumour type	Management
• Local removable (+/– local LN involvement)	Curative surgery
• Local irremovable	DXT
• Local irremovable obstructing/complicating	Palliative surgery, stenting, etc.
• Disseminated	Palliative

★Usually comprises surgery, DXT, chemotherapy (e.g. leukaemia/lymphoma).
★★Usually comprises surgery, DXT, chemotherapy, hormone manipulation (breast, prostate), pain relief, terminal nursing care.

Prognosis depends on:

> **Pathology**
> - Micro – grade: differentiation well, moderate, poor and anaplastic
> - Spread – stage: TNM, oestrogen receptors, etc. – perivascular/neural invasion
>
> **General condition of the patient**
>
> **Anatomical situation**
> - Ca rectum in a male may be inoperable whereas it may be operable in a female
> - Ca oesophagus   lower third >> upper third
> - Malignant melanoma • 25%   0%   5YS

Follow up will depend on the possibilities of recurrence or relapse

PRINCIPLES OF OPERATIVE SURGERY[15]

These can be broken down into:

Preoperative

- Emergency/planned
- Obtain informed consent (any unusual outcomes)
- Mark the site
- Special investigations – cross-matching
- Special preparations – bowel
- Antibiotic prophylaxis and steroid cover
- DVT prophylaxis
- Tubes

Preincision

- Anaesthesia and monitoring
- Position of patient
- Skin preparation
- Position of surgeon
- Incision

Procedure

- The approach (anatomy)
- The procedure
- Recognized problems
- Check haemostasis
- Swab and instrument count
- Closure

Postoperative management

- Timings – sutures, drains, tubes, dressings
- Monitor progress
- Specific instructions
- Specific investigations
- Recognized complications

Follow up and discharge

Complications can be classified as:
- Medical, anaesthetic, surgical

or
- Preoperative, intra-operative, postoperative

or
- Early and late, general and specific

or
- By systems:
    - Mental
    - Cardiac (including haemorrhage)
    - Respiratory
    - Gastrointestinal
    - Urological
    - Locomotor
    - Epidermal
    - Metabolic
    - Infective

Examples of early and late postoperative complications

Early (day 1)
- Haemorrhage – primary or reactive
- Shock – haemorrhagic, cardiogenic, septic
- Oliguria
- Urinary retention
- Pain
- Paralytic ileus
- Atelectasis

Thereafter
- Pyrexia wound
- i.v. line
- Pneumonia
- UTI
- Intra-abdominal sepsis
- DVT
- Pulmonary embolus
- Confusion
- Infection
- Drugs
- Alcohol
- Electrolytes
- Organ failure
- Urinary retention
- Psychiatric

Late
- Adhesions
- Incisional hernias
- Recurrence of original disease

For specific general/local go through systems (see above) or surgical sieve.

1

THE SURGICAL PATIENT

PREOPERATIVE ASSESSMENT[34]

The preoperative evaluation of patients aims to reduce the morbidity and mortality associated with surgery and anaesthesia.

Aim of preoperative planning

- Inform patient of the proposed procedure
- Obtain informed consent for proposed procedure
- Assess pre-existing conditions and estimate their impact on physiological reserve
- Plan postoperative management of these conditions
- Plan analgesia

Issues that should be discussed with a patient preoperatively[28]

- Preoperative medication
- Transport time to operating theatre
- Sequence of events prior to induction of anaesthesia
- Anticipated duration of surgery
- Description of where awakening will occur
- Presence of catheters, lines or bags on awakening
- Expected time of return to hospital ward
- Likelihood of postoperative nausea and vomiting
- Magnitude of postoperative pain and treatment
- Whether they will receive any blood transfusions, with associated risks

Important coexisting medical diseases and increase the morbidity and mortality of surgery[14]

- Ischaemic heart disease
- Congestive cardiac failure
- Hypertension
- Cardiac arrhythmias
- Atrial fibrillation
  - Atrial flutter
  - Atrioventricular block
  - Intraventricular conduction defects
- Chronic respiratory disease
  - Asthma
  - Chronic bronchitis and emphysema
  - Smoking
- Diabetes mellitus
  - Blood disorders
  - Anaemia
  - Haemoglobinopathies
- Others
  - Endocrine dysfunction
  - Renal disease
  - Chronic renal failure
  - Nephrotic syndrome
  - Hepatocellular disease
  - Obstructive jaundice

Non-specific factors that may increase the operative risk for patients undergoing surgery

- Age >70 years
- Surgery >3 h
- Elective versus emergency operation
- Presence of associated illnesses
- Physiological reserve impaired
- Infection risk increased: age, obesity, malnutrition, diabetes (especially uncontrolled), immunosuppression, cancer; radiotherapy, steroid use; insertion of foreign bodies
- Long interval between shaving of operative site and surgery

Preoperative assessment of fitness for anaesthesia and surgery[34]

Cardiovascular system investigations:

- *Chest X-ray*: identifies cardiomegaly and venous congestion associated with cardiac failure.
- *ECG*: a normal resting ECG does not exclude the presence of ischaemic heart disease. However, in the absence of symptoms and signs of coronary disease, there is good correlation between a normal resting ECG and an uneventful preoperative course.
- *Stress ECGs*: show a significant correlation with the development of preoperative complications in patients who:
  - show ischaemic changes during exercise; and
  - are unable to reach 85% of their predicted maximum heart rate during exercise
- *Isotopic scanning*: thallium scanning can determine the ventricular ejection fraction. An ejection fraction <0.30 correlates with significantly increased risk of preoperative myocardial infarction.
- *Echocardiography*: can detect abnormalities of the ventricular wall and assess ventricular contractility.
- *Coronary angiography*: provides definitive evidence of the degree and extent of coronary occlusion and is essential before coronary bypass surgery.

CARDIAC SYSTEM

MAJOR CARDIAC RISK FACTORS

- Myocardial infarction within previous 3 (major risk) or 6 (moderate risk) months
- Unstable angina
- Untreated cardiac failure
- Significant aortic valve stenosis
- Untreated hypertension

RELATIVE CARDIAC RISK FACTORS

- Prior myocardial infarction
- Jugular vein distension (or S1 gallop)
- Non-sinus rhythm
- Ventricular ectopic beats/min
- Age >70 years
- Surgery >3 h

- Emergency surgery
- Significant medical impairment
- P_aO_2 <60 mmHg; P_aCO_2 >50 mmHg
- Chronic liver impairment

Postoperative cardiac complications result from an impaired physiological reserve and being unable to cope with the stresses of the operative period, e.g.:

- Myocardial depression from sepsis and anaesthetic agents.
- Variable pre- and after-load because of fluid shifts associated with disease, surgery and fluid replacement regimens.
- Reduction in oxygen transport due to myocardial depression, intrapulmonary shunting, blood loss and pain- or drug-induced hypoventilation.
- Miscellaneous factors such as hypotension, acidosis, tachycardia, fluctuating blood levels of therapeutic agents.

Myocardial infarction

- Prior myocardial infarction carries an increased rate of reinfarction. The mortality rate from perioperative myocardial infarction is high (40–60%). Thus elective surgery should not be performed within 6 months of myocardial infarction.

Previous pathology	Associated risk of myocardial infarction
No previous infarction	5%
Acute myocardial infarction >6 months previously	6%
Myocardial infarction 3-6 months ago	10-15%
Infarction <3 months ago	30%

Angina

- The clinical assessment of the severity of angina may be based on the grading system devised by the New York Heart Association.

Assessment of angina	Investigation	Risk of surgery
Class 1: Angina with strenuous exercise	Exercise ECG	None
Class 2: Angina with moderate exercise	Exercise ECG	None
Class 3: Angina after climbing one flight of stairs or walking one block	Coronary angiography and coronary artery surgery	High incidence of myocardial infarct
Class 4: Angina with any exercise	Prior to elective surgery	High incidence of myocardial infarct

Hypertension

- WHO df: a systolic blood pressure >160 mmHg and/or a diastolic blood pressure >95 mmHg.
- Mild controlled hypertension poses no additional operative risk but uncontrolled hypertension has a 30% risk of congestive cardiac failure or myocardial infarction in the preoperative period. Elective surgery should be curtailed if the diastolic blood pressure >115 mmHg as a diastolic blood pressure >120 mmHg has a well-documented association with preoperative complications.

Pre- and postoperative aims

- Assessment and optimization of blood pressure control.
- Assessment of associated pathology: coronary disease, congestive failure, renal dysfunction, peripheral vascular disease and coronary disease.
- Anaesthetic management: accurate monitoring of blood pressure, management of intubation hypertension and observation of intraoperative hypertension or signs of ischaemia.
- Postoperative management: optimise pain control and blood pressure management prior to return or oral medication.

RESPIRATORY SYSTEM

Patients at risk of postoperative pulmonary complications[5]

Condition	Mechanism
Obesity	Reduced functional residual capacity
Chronic obstructive airways disease	Secretional airway obstruction from bronchorrhoea and absence of ciliary activity
Chronic smokers	Secretional airway obstruction from bronchorrhoea, diminishes ciliary activity, carboxyhaemoglobinaemia
Restricted airways disease	Diminished vital capacity
Elderly and enfeebled	Aspiration

ASSESSMENT OF RESPIRATORY FUNCTION

- Clinical estimation of the forced expiratory volume in 1 s (FEV1) gives a good index of the severity of airways obstruction.
- Accompanying the patient during stair climbing verifies the degree of exertional dyspnoea.
- Ability to count beyond 20 at a single inspiration further quantifies dyspnoea.

Laboratory testing accurately quantities the degree of impairment as well as recording effects of therapy such as bronchodilator administration. The commonest tests are:

- Spirometry: measures the volumes of exhaled gas per unit time (Figure 1.1). The commonly assessed parameters are:
  - Forced vital capacity (FVC)
  - FEV1

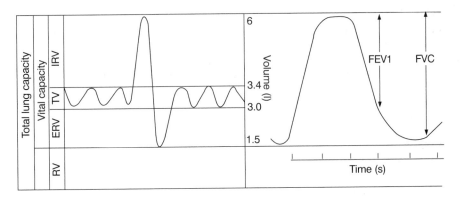

Figure 1.1 Basic spirometry. RV = Residual volume; ERV = expiratory reserve volume; TV = tidal volume; IRV = inspiratory reserve volume; FEV1 = forced expiratory capacity in 1 second; FVC = forced vital capacity.

- FEV/FVC ratio: usually >85%; <50% indicates that postoperative ventilation is more likely; and
- Maximum mid-expiratory flow rate (MMEFR)
- Peak expiatory flow rate (PEFR) measures airflow obstruction at high flow rates.
- Arterial blood gas estimation provides information as to baseline levels of gas transfer and helps guide therapy.

Significant risk factors of postoperative respiratory failure

- Respiratory rate >40/min
- P_aCO_2 >50 mmHg
- P_aO_2 <60 mmHg
- Gradient >300 mmHg on 100% oxygen
- $V_d/V_t = 0.6$
- FVC <15 ml/kg
- FEV1 <45% predicted value

Risk factors which increase the incidence of postoperative pulmonary complications

History
- Preoperative symptoms of respiratory disease
- Preoperative history of chronic obstructive airways disease
- Preoperative productive cough
- Cigarette smoking
- Poor nutrition
- Age >60 years

Examination
- Obesity
- Abnormal chest examination
- Abnormal chest X-ray

Surgery and anaesthesia
- Thoracic and upper abdominal surgery
- Anaesthesia >3 h

Techniques that reduce the incidence of postoperative pulmonary complications

- Bronchodilator therapy
- Pre- and postoperative chest physiotherapy
- Optimal analgesia
- Cessation of smoking 68 weeks prior to major surgery
- Use of the incentive spirometer as an adjunct to physiotherapy
- Early ambulation
- Prophylactic antibiotics if chest infection is present

Chronic obstructive airways disease (COAD)

- COAD includes a group of destructive lung diseases characterized by dyspnoea of progressive severity, airflow obstruction and cough, leading to hypoxaemia and hypercarbia. Intercurrent chest infections are common and right ventricular dysfunction is seen in up to 50% of patients with COAD.
- To quantitate the level of impairment. FEV1 is the most commonly used although the MMEFR is more sensitive. The response to β_2 selective agonists such as salbutamol should be ascertained prior to surgery.
- COAD patients can desaturate during sleep and this may contribute to the incidence of myocardial infarction in the early postoperative days. Physiotherapy commencing preoperatively significantly improves the outcome, especially in patients with significant sputum production.

Asthma

- Asthma is a syndrome of heightened bronchial reactivity resulting in airflow obstruction of variable severity. The overall incidence in the population is 4%.

Assessment of an asthma patient

- Respiratory function test: Spirometry should be performed to asses FVC and FEV1 and allows assessment of the response to bronchodilators.
- Preoperative aim: Optimization of drug therapy and estimation of baseline respiratory function, allowing grading of severity of asthma:

Type	Treatment
Mild asthma (no previous hospitalization)	Maintain routine therapy and administer selective β_2-agonist (salbutamol) via aerosol or nebulizer prior to surgery
Moderate asthma (some functional impairment, routine use of bronchodilators)	Maintain routine therapy and administer selective β_2-agonist (salbutamol) prior to surgery
Severe asthma (significant impairment, current bronchoconstriction)	Corticosteroids should be used (e.g. hydrocortisone 13 mg/kg) 2 h prior to surgery in addition to inhaled β_2-agonist therapy

RENAL SYSTEM

Associated medical problems of patients with chronic renal failure

Cardiovascular
- Hypertension and associated complications
  - Chronic anaemia★ due to ureamia and reduced erythoropoietin levels

Acid–base and metabolic
- Metabolic acidosis
- Hyperkalaemia★★
- Hypocalcaemia
- Hypermagnesaemia
- Inability to manage a water load

Immune system
- Concurrent use of immunosuppressants
- Decreased phagocyte effectiveness

Coagulation
- Coagulopathy: reduced platelet adhesiveness

Presence of an arterovenous fistula
- Problems with venous access
- Limited blood pressure monitoring sites
- Maintenance of fistula function during anaesthesia and recovery

Miscellaneous
- Delayed gastric emptying (uraemia)
- Associated diabetes
- Altered drug metabolism: muscle relaxants, pethidine, aminoglycosides

ENDOCRINE SYSTEM

Diabetes

- Incidence ~2.5% of the population have diabetes >90% have non-insulin-dependent diabetes mellitus (NIDDM or Type II diabetes).

Assessment of coexistent problems

- Cardiovascular system: microvascular disease is widespread and is frequently associated with left ventricular dysfunction. Between 15 and 60% of insulin-dependent diabetics having ECG changes.
- Hypertension: present in >60% of diabetic patients. Orthostatic hypotension is a reliable indicator of the presence of autonomic neuropathy, an uncommon but serious complication of diabetes with impaired cardiovascular responses to exercise and stress.
- Peripheral vascular disease: with the risk of vascular occlusion during periods of hypotension or hypovolaemia.
- Renal disease: glomerulosclerosis, papillary necrosis and ultimately chronic renal failure.

★ Haemoglobin levels of 7-10 g/l are normal in patients with chronic renal failure and injudicious transfusion may result in the precipitation of cardiac failure.
★★Serum potassium should be reduced to between 5.5 and 6.0 mmol/l prior to surgery by dialysis, glucose–insulin therapy or resonium enemas. Suxamethonium, administration of blood and hypoventilation may all increase serum potassium.

Preoperative preparation of the diabetic[14,28]

Type of diabetes	Type of surgery	
	Minor	**Immediate/major**
Controlled by diet	No specific precautions	Measure blood glucose 4-hourly: if > 12 mmol/l start dextrose-insulin infusion. Avoid i.v. dextrose
Controlled by oral agents	Omit medication on morning of operation and start when eating normally postoperatively	Onit medication and monitor blood glucose 1–2 hourly: if > 12 mmol/l start dextrose-insulin infusion
Controlled by insulin	Unless very minor procedure (omit insulin when nil by mouth) give dextrose-insulin infusion during surgery and until eating normally postoperatively	

Hypothyroidism

Affects an estimated 3-5% of the population and is frequently subclinical. Hypothyroid patients are very sensitive to anaesthetic and sedative agents and consequently have an increased need for respiratory support postoperatively and should be rendered euthyroid preoperatively.

Hyperthyroidism

Hyperthyroid patients should be rendered euthyroid before surgery using β-blockade and antithyroid drugs (propylthiouracil or similar).

Complications that may occur during the perioperative period in patients with uncontrolled hyperthyroidism include:

- Thyroid storm, which is an acute episode of profound thyroid hyperactivity associated with tachycardia, pyrexia and cardiac arrhythmias. (If untreated, this condition has a high mortality rate)
- Precipitation of angina, myocardial infarction or cardiac failure
- Tachyarrhythmias
- Treatment in emergency surgery use:
  - Intravenous administration of antithyroid drugs
  - Indwelling arterial monitoring
  - Sedating premedication to allay anxiety
  - Avoidance of drugs that may provoke tachycardia, such as ketamine, pancuronium and atropine
  - Use of β-blockade to control heart rate
  - Adequate depth of anaesthesia to ablate noxious stimuli
  - Good postoperative pain control

OTHER INFLUENCES ON ANAESTHETIC RISK

Alcohol

Potential perioperative problems:

- Cellular tolerance leading to higher anaesthetic requirements
- Chronic brain syndrome (alcoholic dementia)
- Clotting abnormalities
- Increased risk of infection
- Poor wound healing
- Acute withdrawal syndrome (delerium tremens)
- Agitation and self-harm
- Wound disruption
- Cardiovascular instability
- Bleeding varices

Smoking

No decrease in postoperative complications has been found unless smoking is stopped >8 weeks prior to surgery.

Concurrent drug treatment

- Steroids: use of oral steroids for >2 weeks in the preceding 9 months may cause adrenal suppression. Oral steroid supplementation during the perioperative period should be used in patients suspected of being at risk.
- Immunosuppressants: prolong effect of suxamethonium, increase the risk of wound infection and delay wound healing.
- Tricyclic antidepressants: antidepressants should only be discontinued in consultation with the treating psychiatrist.
- Monoamine oxidase inhibitors: following consultation with the treating psychiatrist, monoamine oxidase inhibitors (MAOI) should be discontinued 2-3 weeks prior to surgery to allow regeneration of adequate levels of monoamine oxidase.

Guidelines on MAOI:

- Preoperative consultation with the treating psychiatrist.
- Benzodiazepine premedication.
- Avoid halothane, pethidine.
- If vasopressors are necessary, avoid indirect-acting pressors (metaraminol) and use fluids and posture wherever possible. Carefully titrate small doses of direct-acting vaso-constrictors (methoxamine or phenylephrine) if necessary.
- Suxamethonium: effect may be prolonged due to decreased cholinesterase levels.

Oral contraceptives

- The progesterone-only pill poses no documented problems during surgery.
- The combination oestrogen–progesterone pill should be discontinued 6 weeks prior to elective surgery because of the increased risk of deep vein thrombosis (DVT), especially in women who smoke. When emergency surgery is necessary, additional thomboembolism prophylaxis is required. The patient must be advised to use alternate forms of contraception as the reliability of oral absorption is affected by fasting, perioperative nausea and vomiting and any antibiotic-induced diarrhoea.

11

Prophylaxis of thromboembolic disease

- Clinically significant but non-fatal thromboembolism occurs in about 1:100 postoperative patients and fatal pulmonary embolism in 1:1000 (see page XX for the definition of high-risk groups plus prophylaxis and treatment).

ADVANTAGES OF PRE-ADMISSION CLINICS[34]

- Reduction in bed occupancy and thus a shorter hospital stay
- Less disruption to patient's routine
- Development of guidelines for laboratory investigations means that appropriate tests are performed and unnecessary laboratory tests are minimized
- Adequate time exists between consultation and surgery for the relevant tests to be performed and the results obtained
- Fewer 'last minute' cancellations because of abnormal test results

ROUTINE INVESTIGATION PRIOR TO SURGERY[34]

Routine preoperative tests for asymptomatic patients		
Age (years)	Male	Female
0–12	–	–
12–39	–	Hb (or Hct)
40–49	ECG	Hb/Hct
50–64	ECG	Hct, ECG
65+	Hct, Hb, ECG, BUN, glucose	Hb (Hct), ECG, BUN, glucose

Biochemistry

Significant previously undetected abnormalities occur in <1% of cases. Liver function tests are only indicated when clinically detectable disease is present. Routine biochemical testing is not indicated on asymptomatic patients <60 years of age.

Haematology

The lowest acceptable level of haemoglobin in most studies is 7 g/dl (when major blood loss is not anticipated). Chronic anaemia (Hb <9 g/l) should be corrected prior to elective surgery as the patient will have reduced reserve to compensate for intraoperative blood loss. Routine coagulation screening should only be done when clinically indicated or when undetected coagulopathy would be a major problem, such as in neurosurgery and heart surgery. Sickle cell status should be determined in patients at risk.

Chest X-ray

- A chest X-ray should be performed only to confirm a suspected pathological condition likely to affect outcome from surgery, e.g.:
  - Pulmonary metastases and mediastinal masses
  - Tuberculosis
  - Significant lung disease, e.g. pneumonia, pulmonary oedema or atelectasis
  - Thoracic pathology such as fractured ribs, pneumothorax or pleural fluid accumulation

ECG

Abnormalities on routine ECG are found in 50% of cases but rarely (1.6%) cause postoperative problems. However, the ECG may provide the only indication of recent myocardial infarction. An ECG should be performed on all patients with known cardiovascular disease and on asymptomatic patients >40 years of age.

Clinically 'silent' conditions detectable on ECG screening that will alter perioperative management:

- Atrial flutter or fibrillation
- Left or right ventricular hypertrophy
- Conduction problems: heart block, Wolff–Parkinson–White syndrome, ischaemia, myocardial infarction, pulmonary embolism, atrial or ventricular ectopics, prolonged 'QT' interval

Pulmonary function tests

Spirometry should be performed on patients with dyspnoea on mild-to-moderate exertion (see **Figure 1.1**).

FLUID BALANCE

Average daily water balance for sedentary adult in temperate conditions[14]				
Input	**(ml)**	**Output**	**(ml)**	
Drink	1500	Urine	1500	
Food	750	Faeces	100	
Metabolic	350	Lungs	400	
		Skin	600	
Total	**2600**	**Total**	**2600**	

Electrolyte content and daily volume of body secretion[14]				
	Na (mmol/l)	**K (mmol/l)**	**Cl (mmol/l)**	**Volume (litres/day)**
Saliva	15	19	40	1.5
Stomach	50	15	140	2.5
Bile, pancreas, small bowel	130–145	5–12	70–100	4.2
Insensible sweat	12	10	12	0.6
Sensible sweat	50	10	50	variable

The normal daily (hourly) fluid requirement to replace insensible losses and produce modest diuresis is		
First 10 kg	100 ml/kg	(4 ml/kg)
Second 10 kg	50 ml/kg	(2 ml/kg)
Each subsequent kg	20 ml/kg	(1 ml/kg)

Initial management of oliguria in the surgical patient[14]

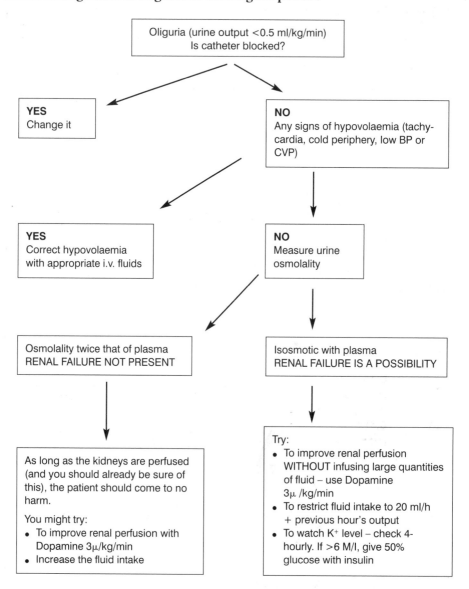

Changes resulting from three kinds of expansion and contraction of body fluids[14] note change in haematocrit (Hct)

Acute Change	Example	Change in ECF vol.	Change in ICF vol.	Change in Na	Change in Hct
Loss of H_2O+NACl	Cholera	↓	→	→	↑
Loss of H_2O>Na	XS Sweating	↓	↓	↑	→
Loss of Na>H_2O	Addisons	↓	↑	↓	↑
Isotonic expansion	Saline Infusion	↑	→	→	↓
Hypertonic expansion	2 x Normal Saline	↑	↑	↓	→
Hypertonic expansion	5% Glucose Infusion	↑	↑	↓	→

Content of crystallised solutions[14]

Name	Contents	Na^+	Cl^-	K^+	HCO_3^-	Ca^{2+}	Calculated mosmol/l
Normal saline	Sodium chloride 0.9%	150	150	–			300
Normal saline + KCl	Sodium chloride 0.9% Potassium chloride 0.3%	150	190	40			380
Normal saline + KCl	Sodium chloride 0.9% Potassium chloride 0.15%	150	170	20			340
Hartmann's	Ringer's lactate	131	111	5	29*		280
5% dextrose	Glucose 5%	–	–	–			280
5% dextrose + KCl	Glucose 5% Potassium chloride 0.3%	–	40	40			360
5% dextrose + KCl	Glucose 5% Potassium chloride 0.15%	–	20	20			320
Dextrose saline	Glucose 4% Sodium chloride 0.18%	–	30	30			286
Dextrose saline + KCl	Glucose 4% Sodium chloride 0.18% Potassium chloride 0.3%	–	30	70	40		366
Dextrose saline + KCl	Glucose 4% Sodium chloride 0.18% Potassium chloride 0.15%	–	30	50	20		326

* 12 as lactate

Name	Contents	Na⁺	Cl⁻	K⁺	HCO₃⁻	Ca²⁺	Calculated mosmol/l
Half normal saline	Sodium chloride 0.45%	–	75	75			150
Twice normal saline	Sodium chloride 1.8%	–	300	300			600
Sodium bicarbonate 8.4%		–	1000	1000			2000
Sodium bicarbonate 1.4%		–	167	167			334

Characteristics of colloid solutions[14]

Name	Brand names	No. av. mol. wt*	Mol. wt range	Na⁺	K⁺	Ca²⁺	Half life in plasma	Adverse reactions (%) Mild	Severe	Effect on coagulation
Human plasma protein factor	HPPF	69 000	69 000	150	5	2	20 days	0.02	0.004	None
Dextran 70 in saline 0.9% or glucose 5%	Macro-dex Lomo-dex 70 Gentran 70	38 000	10 000–250 000	150	–	–	12 h	0.7	0.02	Inhibit platelet aggregations Factor VIII↓ Interfere with crossmatch
Polygeline	Haem-accel	24 500	5 000–50 000	145	5	6.25	2.5 h	0.12	0.04	None (degrade gelatin)
Succinyl-ated gelatin	Gelo-fusion	22 600	10 000–140 000	154	0.4	0.4	4 h	0.12	0.04	None
Hydroxyl-ethyl starch 6% saline (Hetastarch)	Hespan	70 000	10 000–100 000	154	–	–	20 h	0.09	0.006	>1.5 g/kg/day can cause coagulopathy

* Number average molecular weight should not be confused with weight average molecular weight, which is usually quoted by the manufacturers. Number average molecular weight is more appropriate

BLOOD PRODUCTS AND TRANSFUSION

Functions of blood	Component	Minimum of normal required
Maintenance of intravascular volume	Volume	60%
Oxygen carrying capacity	Haemoglobin	50%
Haemostasis	Platelets, coagulation factors	10%
Maintenance of oncotic pressure	Plasma proteins	10%

Use of blood products	
Blood products	**Use**
Whole blood (510 ml)	Major haemorrhage
Packed cells (plasma-reduced blood 280 ml)	Anaemia
Filtered cells (washed red cells)	To avoid transfusion reaction
Platelet concentrate	Thrombocytopenia
Fresh frozen plasma (FFP)	Coagulation disorders (more dilute than the concentrate below)
Cryoprecipitate (rich in factor VIII)	Hypofibrigenaemia, factor XIII, def, von Willebrand disease
Factor II VII VIII, IX, X, XI concentrate	Specific coagulation disorders

Factors that may affect delivery of oxygen to the tissues[14]

- Haemoglobin oxygenation
- Partial pressure of oxygen in air
- Haemoglobin concentration
- Haemoglobin oxygen saturation
- Haemoglobin affinity for oxygen
- Effects of pH, 2,3-DPG and haemoglobins with high affinity for oxygen
- Blood volume
- Cardiac output
- Peripheral vascular resistance
- Lung function
- Type and duration of anaesthesia
- Type and duration of surgery

Main types of anaemia and their management

Type	Management
Anaemia due to decreased production of blood cell	Establish diagnosis, deal with the cause and prescribe oral iron preparation

Iron deficiency anaemia
  Nutritional or due to malabsorption
  Chronic blood loss
	Usually with good response

Vitamin B$_{12}$ deficiency	Establish diagnosis, deal with the cause and treat with parenteral vitamin B12
Nutritional or due to malabsorption Pernicious anaemia	Usually with good response
Folic acid deficiency	Establish diagnosis, deal with the cause and prescribe folic acid.
Usually nutritional or due to malabsorption	With a good response
Anaemia of chronic disease	Establish diagnosis and treat the primary disease
	Usually poor response
	Patients with renal disease respond to rhEPO*
Anaemia due to bone marrow failure	Establish diagnosis and treat the primary disease.
	Variable response. Transfuse as required.
Aplastic anaemia, leukaemia, bone marrow	Sometimes transfusion of platelets is also needed
infiltration with malignant cells	
Anaemia due to increased destruction of red cells	Establish diagnosis. Transfuse as and when required

Inherited
  Haemoglobinopathies
  Thalassaemia
  Sickle cell disease
	Establish diagnosis and treat the primary disease.

Acquired Immune-mediated Non-immune haemolytic anaemias	Avoid transfusion where possible
Anaemia due to blood loss Acute	Remove cause of bleeding where possible, transfuse where required
Chronic	Manage as iron deficiency anaemia

*rhEPO, recombinant human erythropoietin.

Risks of transfusion

Early

- Immediate haemolytic transfusion reaction: mismatch error
- Delayed haemolytic transfusion reaction: haemolysis of transfused cells
- Non-haemolytic febrile transfusion reaction
- Immunomodulation

- Large transfusions
  - Hypothermia
  - Hypocalcaemia
  - Hyperkalaemia
  - Coagulopathy, DIC
  - Release of vasoactive peptides
  - Release of plasticisers from PVC-phthalates
- Physical complications
  - Circulatory overload
  - Air embolism
  - Pulmonary embolism
  - Thrombophlebitis
  - ARDS

Late

- Transmission of infection
  - Hep B★, Hep C★, HIV★, Treponema pallidum★, cytomegalo-virus (CMV) and Epstein–Barr virus (EBV)
  - Brucellosis, toxoplasmosis, malaria
  - American trypanosomiasis (Chaga's disease)
- Haemosiderosis: after repeated transfusion in patients with haematological disease

Estimates of virus transmission rates by transfusion of blood and blood components[14]

Virus	Incidence of carriers	Tests available	Tests used	Estimate of units required for transfusion
Hepatitis B virus	1:1000	Yes	Yes	20 000
Non-A, non-B viruses	1:1700	Yes	Yes	20 000
Cytomegalovirus	1:2	Yes	No	10
Epstein-Barr virus	9:10	Yes	No	Most recipients are immune
HIV 1 and 2	1:25 000	Yes	Yes	1 000 000
HTLV I and II	1:20 000	Yes	No	1 000 000

Adverse immune reactions of blood transfusion[14]

- Immune response to cellular and plasma alloantigens
  - Clinical syndromes following repeated transfusions
  - Red cell antibodies: haemolytic transfusion reaction
  - HLA antibodies
    - Non-haemolytic febrile transfusion reaction
    - Platelet refractoriness
  - Platelet antibodies
    - Platelet refractoriness
    - Post-transfusion thrombocytopenia
    - Neonatal immune thrombocytopenia
  - Anti-IgA★: anaphylactic shock

★ Routine screening

- Immunomodulation (e.g. reduced disease free interval after resection of carcinoma of the colon)
- Graft-versus-host disease (caused by transfusion of live lymphocytes)
  - In immunosuppressed patients (e.g. patients receiving tissue or organ transplants)
  - In immunocompetent patients (transfused with blood donated by first-degree relatives)

Differential diagnosis of haemostatic failure[14]

Condition or platelet disease	Laboratory tests			
	Prothrombin time	Partial thromboplastin time	Thrombin time	Platelet* count
Massive blood transfusion	+	+	N	–
DIC	++	++	++	– –
Vitamin K deficiency	++	+	N	N
Haemophilias	N	++	N	N
ITP	N	N	N	– –

* Platelet count rarely falls below 50 × 10 l^{-1}
N = normal; + = moderately prolonged; ++ = markedly prolonged;
– = moderately decreased;
– – = markedly decreased
DIC = disseminated intravascular coagulation
ITP = idiopathic thrombocytopenic purpura

NUTRITION

BASIC PATIENT NUTRITIONAL REQUIREMENTS[5]

Daily requirement per kg body weight:
- Water – 30–50 ml
- Calories – 30–50 kcal
- Nitrogen – 0.20–0.35 g
- Sodium – 0.9–1.2 mmol
- Potassium – 0.7–0.9 mmol

CLINICAL STAGING OF MALNUTRITION AND METHODS OF MONITORING[29]

Clinical/lab parameters	Extent of malnutrition		
	Mild	Moderate	Severe
Albumin	28~32	21~27	<21
Transferrin (mg/dl)	200–250	100–200	<100
Total lymphocyte count	1200–2000	800–1200	<800
Ideal body weight (%)	80–90	70–80	<70
Usual body weight (%)	85–95	75–85	<75
Weight loss/unit time	<5% per month >10% over 6 months	<2% per week >5% per month >10%/ 6/12	>2% per week >5% per month

ROUTES OF ADMINISTRATION FOR NUTRITION[14]

Enteral
- Oral feeding
- Tube feeding
- Nasoenteral
- Gastric, duodenal or jejunal
- Cervical pharyngostomy
- Cervical oesophagostomy
- Gastrostomy
  - Surgical or percutaneous endoscopic gastrostomy (PEG)
- Jejunostomy
  - Surgical or needle catheter jejunostomy (NCJ)

Parenteral

CATEGORIES OF PATIENTS SUITABLE FOR ENTERAL NUTRITION[14]

Skin tests	Normal	Weak	Anergic
(Reaction/tests)	4/4	1–2/4	0/4
Normal anthropometric measurements			
	Male	Female	
Triceps skin fold (mm)	12.5	16.5	
Midarm circumference	29.3	28.5	

Note: if severe malnutrition is present nutritional therapy is indicated.

Patient group	Disease state
Medical	Inflammatory bowel disease
	Hepatic failure
	Renal failure
	Respiratory failure
Neurological	Cerebrovascular accident
	Motor neurone disease
	Multiple sclerosis
Geriatric	
Surgical	Preoperative
	Postoperative
	Fistula
	Burns
	Sepsis
Orthopaedic	Trauma
Psychiatric	Anorexia nervosa
Paediatric	Cystic fibrosis
Miscellaneous	ITU
	Cancer
	Short bowel
	AIDS/HIV

COMPLICATIONS OF ENTERAL NUTRITION[14]

Feeding tube related
- Malposition
- Unwanted removal
- Blockage

Diet and administration-related
- Diarrhoea
- Bloating
- Nausea
- Cramps
- Regurgitation
  - Diseases with an increased risk of regurgitation and aspiration include:
    - Diabetes with neuropathy
    - Hypothryroidism
    - ITU patients on ventilators
    - Neuromotor deglutition disorders
    - Neurosurgical patients
- Post-abdominal surgery
- Pulmonary aspiration (see below)
- Vitamin, mineral, trace element deficiencies
- Drug interactions

Metabolic/biochemical

Infective
- Diets
- Reservoirs
- Giving sets

CATEGORIES OF PATIENTS SUITABLE FOR TOTAL PARENTERAL NUTRITION (TPN)[14]

Patient group	Disease state
Medical	Inflammatory bowel disease
	Hepatic failure
	Renal failure
	Respiratory failure
Surgical	Preoperative
	Postoperative
	Burns
	Sepsis
	Pancreatitis
Orthopaedic	Trauma
Miscellaneous	ITU
	Cancer
	Short bowel
	AIDS/HIV

IMPORTANT FACTORS TO CONSIDER BEFORE STARTING TPN[14]

- Access
- Techniques
- Delivery
- Complications
- Nutrients
- Monitoring
- Metabolic complications

TPN REGIMENS[14]

Nutrient	In moderate injury	(ml)	In severe injury	(ml)
Nitrogen*	14 g	1000	17g	1000
Energy glucose*				
Dextrose 50%	1000 kcal	500	1000 kcal	500
Dextrose 20%	400 kcal	500	800 kcal	1000
Lipid				
(20% emulsion)	1000 kcal	500	1000kcal	500
Total volume		**2500**		**3000**

As required: potassium, phosphate, sodium, trace elements, vitamins (water soluble), vitamins (fat soluble), (insulin)

*Differences in nitrogen densities, glucose and lipid concentrations allow manipulation of actual volume.

COMPLICATIONS OF TPN

Complications of central venous catheter[14]

Insertion related

- Air embolism
- Arterial puncture
- Arrhythmias
- Catheter embolism
- Chylothorax
- Haemo/hydropericardium
- Haematoma
- Haemothorax
- Hydro-TPN-othorax
- Malposition
- Neurological injury
- Pneumothorax

Later complications

- Catheter infection sepsis
- Luminal occlusion
- Catheter displacement
- Central venous system

METABOLIC COMPLICATIONS OF TPN[14]

- Hyperglycaemia, hypoglycaemia
- Hypophosphataemia
- Hypercalcaemia
- Hyperkalaemia, hypokalaemia, hypernatraemia, hyponatraemia
- Hyperosmolar diuresis
- Other deficiencies of folate, zinc, magnesium, other trace elements, vitamins and essential fatty acids
- Hepatobiliary dysfunction

ANAESTHETICS

AMERICAN SOCIETY OF ANAESTHESIOLOGISTS' CLASSIFICATION OF PHYSICAL STATUS (ASA)[14]

I – healthy patient
II – mild systemic disease, non functional limitations
III – severe systemic disease with definite functional limitation
IV – severe systemic disease that is a constant threat to life
V – moribund patient not expected to survive 24 hours with or without operation
(E denotes an emergency)

BLOOD GAS ANALYSIS: NORMAL VALUES[14]

pH	7.35–7.45
P_aO_2	75–100 mmHg, 10–13.3 kPa
P_aCO_2	36–44 mmHg, 4.8–6.0 kPa
S_aO_2	95–100%
Base deficit	+2.5
HCO_2	22–26 mm.l^{-1}

GUIDELINES FOR INTRODUCTION OF MECHANICAL VENTILATION[9]

General indications of acute respiratory failure (after Pontoppidan *et al.*)
- Inadequate ventilation
  - Indicated by:
    - Apnoea, upper airway obstruction, unprotected airway
    - Respiratory rate >35 breaths/min (normal range 10–20)
    - Vital capacity <15 ml/kg (normal range 65–75)
    - Tidal volume <5 ml/kg (normal range 5–7)
    - Negative inspiratory force <25 cmH$_2$0 (normal range 75–100)
    - P_aCO_2 >8 kPa (60 mmHg) (normal range 4.7–6.3 kPa (35–47 mmHg)
    - V_d/V_t >0.6 (normal range <0.30)
- Inadequate gas exchange oxygenation
  - Indicated by:
    - P_aO_2 <8 kPa. (60 mmHg) on F_iO_2 > 0.6
    - Alveolar-arterial oxygen gradient (A–) DO$_2$ on F_iO_2 1.0 >47 kPa (350 mmHg) (normal range 3.3–8.7 kPa (25–65 mmHg))

Specific indications, with or without previous respiratory pathology
- Chronic obstructive lung disease
  - Failure of conservative measures
  - Inability to cooperate with care
  - Decreased consciousness
  - Cardiac instability
  - Apnoea
  - Sever respiratory acidosis
  - Acute management of nocturnal obstructive hypoventilation
- Chronic restrictive lung disease
  - Severe hypoxaemia
  - Fatigue and impending exhaustion
- Severe acute asthma
  - Failure of conservative measures
  - Obtundation
  - Cardiac instability
  - Increasing P_aCO_2
  - Fatigue and impending exhaustion
- Head trauma – unconscious, unprotected airway, cerebral oedema, apnoea, or global hypoventilation
- Chest trauma
  - Flail chest with hypoventilation and hypoxaemia
  - Pulmonary contusion with hypoxaemia
- Neuromuscular weakness
  - Apnoea or progressive hypoventilation (see above)
  - Airway protection, nocturnal hypoventilation/hypoxaemia
  - Organophosphate poisoning

- Other neurological disorders – status epilepticus, tetanus, high cervical spine injury
- Upper airway protection
  - Loss of consciousness, neck and oropharyngeal trauma, epiglottitis, acute neuromuscular event
  - Drug overdose
- Apnoea, hypoventilation, airway protection, seizures

MAXIMUM DOSES OF LOCAL ANAESTHETIC AGENTS IN HEALTHY 70 kg ADULT[14]

Agent	Plain solution	With adrenalin
Lignocaine	200 mg (e.g. 20 ml of 1%)	500 mg (e.g. 50 ml of 1%)
Bupivicaine	150 mg (e.g. 30 ml of 0.5%)	200 mg (e.g. 40 ml of 0.5%)
Prilocaine	400 mg (e.g. 80 ml of 1.5%)	600 mg (e.g. 120 ml of 0.5%)

POTENTIAL (PRACTICAL) SITES FOR REGIONAL ANAESTHESIA[35]

Nerve	Digital	Obturator	Ilioinguinal Genitofemoral	Supraorbital
	Median Ulnar	Sciatic Femoral	Dorsal nerve of penis	Intradental
Ganglion	Trigeminal Stellate	Gasserian Lumbar sympathetic		
Plexus	Cervical	Brachial	Coeliac	

RELATIONSHIP BETWEEN SIZE AND FUNCTION OF NERVE FIBRES[35]

Fibre type	Function	Fibre size	Conduction	Onset of block (min)
A Myelinated		Large	Rapid	
α	Somatic proprioception			6
β	Touch			5
γ	Muscle spindle			4
δ	Pain, temperature			3
B Myelinated	Autonomic			1
C Non-myelinated	Pain, temperature	Small	Slow	2

RECOGNITION OF GAS CYLINDERS

Gas	Characteristic
Oxygen	Black body, white collar
Nitrous oxide	French blue body, blue collar
Air	Grey body, black-and-white quartered collar
Entonox (50% nitrous oxide, 50% O_2)	Black body, blue-and-white collar
Carbon dioxide	Grey body with grey collar (not meant to be on anaesthetic machines)

ORGAN FAILURE

CAUSES OF ACUTE RENAL FAILURE[13]

Renal perfusion
- Arterial hypotension
- Decreased systemic vascular resistance (e.g. sepsis)
- Defective renal autoregulation (ACE inhibitors, NSAIDs)
- Hepatorenal syndrome

Renal vasculature
- Renal artery stenosis
- Renal embolism
- Renal arterioles
  - Polyarteritis nodosa
  - Accelerated hypertension
- Glomerular capillaries
  - Goodpastures' syndrome
  - Wegener's disease and microscopic polyarteritis
  - Accelerated hypertension
  - Pre-eclampsia
  - Haemolytic uraemic syndrome
  - Cholesterol embolism
- Renal vein thrombosis

Glomeruli – glomerulonephritis
Tubules
- Intestinal nephritis
- Drug-induced nephrotoxicity
- Contrast nephropathy
- Urate nephropathy
- Acute tubular necrosis

GENERAL MANAGEMENT OF ACUTE RENAL FAILURE[13]

- Correction of hyperkalaemia
- Aggressive correction of hypovolaemia and/or hypotension
- Treatment of underlying cause

- Avoidance of further insults to renal circulation, e.g.
  - Hypotension
  - Hypovolaemia
  - Sepsis
- Avoidance of potentially nephrotic agents where possible
  - Aminoglycosides
  - NSAIDs
  - Contrast media
- Adequate nutrition – enteral and parenteral
- Good nursing care, e.g. prevention of pressure sores
- Correction of uraemia by dialysis
- Full explanation and reassurance

PRACTICAL MANAGEMENT OF ACUTE RENAL FAILURE[13]

- Weigh daily to ensure stable fluid balance
  - Check:
    - Jugular venous pressure and presence or absence of peripheral oedema
    - Lying and standing blood pressure
    - Daily serum electrolytes
  - Careful measurement of fluid input and output
- Intravenous access – central venous pressure line where necessary
- Fluid balance – patients may be hypervolaemic, normovolaemic, or hypovolaemic
  - Normovolaemic
    - If possible give fluids by mouth or by nasogastric tube, otherwise i.v.
    - Maintain balance by daily intake of 300–500 ml plus amount equal to total fluid output on previous day (i.e. urine, stools, vomit, fistula drainage)
  - Hypervolaemic
    - Indicated by an increase in weight, rise in jugular venous pressure or development of peripheral oedema
    - Give no fluid with only minimal fluid for parenteral drugs (usually 5% glucose)
    - Trial of frusemide 180 mg i.v. or 500–1000 mg orally
    - If no diuresis and clinical evidence of pulmonary congestion use ultrafiltration or dialysis
  - Hypovolaemic
    - Indicated by an excessive fall in weight or postural hypotension
    - Replace fluid quickly with normal saline or appropriate fluid

SEPSIS

Sepsis (**Figures 1.2 and 1.3**) is defined as the development of a systemic inflammatory response syndrome (SIRS) as a result of an infective process. It is characterised by two or more of the following conditions:

- Temperature >38.4°C or <35.6°C
- Heart rate >90 beats/min
- Respiratory rate >20 breaths/min or $PaCO_2$ <32 mmHg
- White cell count >12 000 per ml or <4000 cells per ml or 10% immature (band) forms

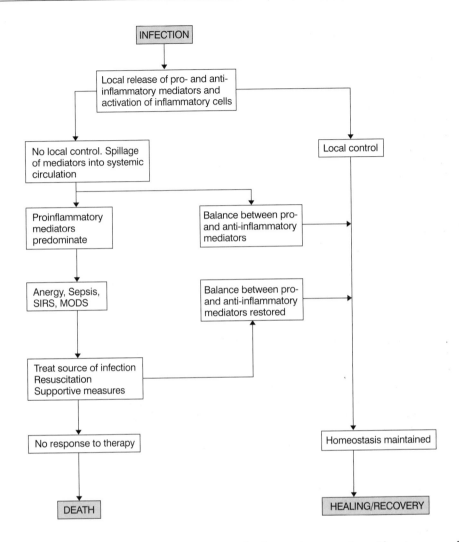

Figure 1.2 Local and systemic response to infection and progression either to successful resolution or deterioration/death. SIRS = systemic inflammatory response syndrome; MODS = multiple organ sysfunction syndrome.

CLINICAL FEATURES OF THE SEPSIS SYNDROME[9]

- Evidence of fever or shock
  - Fever >38°C or hypothermia <36.6°C core temperature
  - Tachycardia >90 beats/min
  - Tachypnoea >20 breaths/min or requiring mechanical ventilation
  - Hypotension, systolic blood pressure <90 mmHg or >40 mmHg fall in systolic pressure, with adequate fluid filing
  - Evidence of localized focus of infection

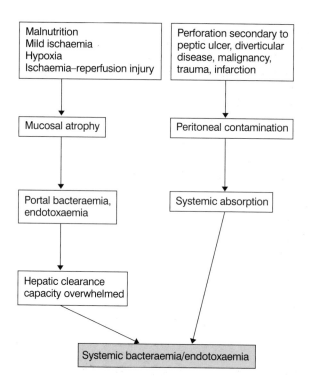

Figure 1.3 Disruption of the mucosal barrier leading to development of systemic toxaemia and endotoxaemia.

- Together with other clinical evidence of toxicity or end-organ failure
  - Metabolic acidosis, pH <7.3 corrected for PCO_2 changes, or a base deficit >5
  - Arterial hypoxaemia with PO_2 <10 kPa
  - $P_aO_2{:}F_iO_2$ ratio >33 (P_aO_2 in kPa) or 250 (P_aO_2 in mmHg)
  - Increased plasma lactate
  - Oliguria <0.5 ml/kg.h for 1 h
  - Coagulation defect with prothrombin time 1.5 times control or PTT 1.2 times control
  - Thrombocytopenia <100 000 or >50% fall within 24 h
  - Acute deterioration in mental status
  - Any other sign of organ system failure

CRITERIA FOR THE PRESENCE OF ORGAN SYSTEM FAILURE[9]

- Circulatory failure
  - Bradycardia (rate <50 beats/min)
  - Hypotension (Mean BP <50 mmHg)
  - Ventricular tachycardia or fibrillation
  - Metabolic acidosis (pH <7.2)

- Respiratory failure
  - Respiratory rate <5 or >40 breaths/min
  - Hypercapnoea ($P_a CO_2$ >6.7 kPa or 50 mmHg)
  - Hypoxaemia ([A–a] PO_2 gradient >50 kPa or 350 mmHg)
- Acute renal failure
  - Urine output <400 ml/24 h or <150 ml/8 h
  - Rising serum creatinine >150 mmol/l
- Haematologic failure
  - Leucopenia (WBC <1000 cells/mm^3)
  - Thrombocytopenia (platelets <20 000/mm^3)
  - Evidence of disseminated intravascular coagulation
- Hepatic failure
  - Coagulation defect (INR >2.0)
  - Rising hepatic enzymes
  - Rising alkaline phosphatase
- Gastrointestinal failure
  - Ileus
  - Gastroparesis
  - Haemorrhage
- Neurological failure
  - Depressed consciousness (Glasgow coma score <6)
  - Seizure disorder

MANAGEMENT OVERVIEW OF ORGAN SYSTEM FAILURE[9]

- Circulatory failure ★
  - Optimise cardiac preload
  - Maximize cardiac contractility with inotropes
  - Maintain perfusion pressures with vasopressors
  - Correct anaemia
  - Treat arrhythmias
- Respiratory failure★
  - Oxygen
  - Mechanical ventilation
  - PEEP/CPAP
  - Extra- and intracorporeal gas exchange
- Acute renal failure
  - Haemofiltration/haemodialysis or:
  - Conservative measures
    - Fluid restriction
    - Potassium restriction
    - Appropriate nitrogen intake
  - Drug dose adjustment
- Haematologic failure
  - Red cell and platelet transfusion
  - Fresh frozen plasma (INR <1.5)
  - Correct antithrombin III deficiency
- Hepatic failure
  - Fresh frozen plasma

- Appropriate nutritional support
- Correct hypoalbuminaemia
- Gastrointestinal failure
  - Parenteral nutrition
  - Stress ulcer prophylaxis
  - Selective decontamination
- Neurological failure – control seizures

* Optimization of circulatory and respiratory parameters to achieve the following therapeutic goals:

- Increased mean blood pressure to 75% premorbid levels
- Increased cardiac index >4.5 l/min.m^2
- Increased oxygen delivery to >600 ml/min.m^2
- Increased oxygen consumption to 170 ml/min.m^2

This should lead to:

- Reduced blood lactate and correction of metabolic acidosis
- Urine output >0.5 ml/kg.h

2

COMPLICATIONS OF SURGERY

MAIN RISK FACTORS FOR COMPLICATIONS IN SURGERY

- Age
- Obesity
- Cardiovascular disease (systemic diseases)
- Respiratory disease
- Diabetes (metabolic disease)
- Drug therapy – steroids, antibiotics, cytotoxics, cyclosporin
- Blood transfusion – incompatibility, storage, disease transmission, altered immunity
- Pathology – obstructive jaundice, uraemia, neoplastic disease
- Type of surgery – orthopaedic, gynaecological
- Radiation

EXAMPLES OF POSTOPERATIVE COMPLICATIONS BY SYSTEMS[10]

- Haemorrhage
  - Early postoperative
  - Secondary haemorrhage
- Wound
  - Infection
  - Bleeding
  - Haematoma
  - Seroma
  - Suture sinus
  - Breakdown (burst abdomen, incisional hernia, anastomotic breakdown: peritonitis, abscess, fistula)
- Cardiovascular
  - Cardiac arrest
  - MI
  - Pulmonary oedema
  - Arrhythmias
  - DVT
- Lung
  - Atelectasis
  - Aspiration
  - Pneumonia
  - PE
  - Pulmonary oedema
  - Pneumothorax
  - ARDS
- Cerebral
  - Confusion (sepsis, electrolyte/gluose, hypoxia, alcohol withdrawal)
  - Stroke
- Urinary
  - Acute retention
  - UTI
  - Acute renal failure
- Gastrointestinal
  - Paralytic ileus
  - Mechanical obstruction

- Acute gastric dilatation
- Constipation
- Other – pressure sores

CONDITIONS AND COMPLICATIONS ASSOCIATED WITH OBESITY[13]

- Psychological
- Osteoarthritis
- Varicose veins
- Hiatus hernia
- Gallstones
- Postoperative problems
- Back strain
- Accident proneness

- Hypertension
- Breathlessness
- Ischaemic heart disease
- Stroke
- Diabetes mellitus
- Hyperlipidaemia
- Menstrual abnormalities

Non-infectious causes	Pulmonary atelectasis
	Dehydration
	Drug fever (including anaesthetics)
	Malignant hyperthermia
	Neoplasms
	Pancreatitis
	Thrombophlebitis
	Tissue trauma
	Transfusion reaction
Infectious causes	Abscess
	Blood stream infection
	Clostridum difficile colitis
	Endocarditis
	Intravenous device infection
	Peritonitis
	Pneumonia
Surgical infection	Superficial incisional infection
	Deep incisional infection
	Space infection
	Transfusion-related infection (cytomegalovirus, hepatitis)
	Urinary tract infection

Figure 2.1 Causes of postoperative fever.

SURGICAL INFECTION

VARIOUS TYPES OF SURGICAL SEPSIS[15]

- Wound infection
- Peritoneal infection
  - Peritonitis
  - Abscess
- Pulmonary infection
- Prosthesis infection
- Septicaemia
- Pseudo membranous colitis

Note: both sources of infection (autogenous or exogenous) need an inoculum of $>10^5$ bacteria.

FACTORS PREDISPOSING TO WOUND INFECTION[15,21]

Host resistance

General factors

- Age
- Obesity
- Malnutrition
- Endocrine and metabolic disorders (diabetes, uraemia and renal insufficiency, jaundice)
- Hypovolaemic shock
- Hypoxia, pulmonary dysfunction
- Anaemia
- Malignant disease
- Immune compromise (corticosteroids, cytotoxic and antimetabolic drugs, AIDS, chemo- and radiotherapy)

Local factors

- Injury related
  - Location
  - Extent
- Poor surgical technique (dead space, haematoma)
- Impaired vascularity/ischaemia
- Haematoma and seroma formation
- Necrotic tissue
- Foreign bodies
- Previous irradiation
- Drainage
- Surgical technique (dead space, haematoma)

Microbial contamination

- Type and virulence of organism
- Size of bacterial inoculum
- Pattern of resistance to antibiotics and antiseptics

Environment related

- Superinfection

- Hygiene
- Long-term ICU stay

PREVENTION OF WOUND INFECTION[21]

- Exogenous
  - Autoclaving
  - Keep staff in theatre to a minimum
  - Skin cleansing of surgical staff
  - Positive pressure ventilation
  - Laminar air flow
  - Treatment of surgical personnel carrying *Staphylococcus aureus*
- Endogenous
  - Skin preparation, e.g. shaving/depilating, antiseptics and adhesive drapes
  - Mechanical bowel preparation (controversial)
  - Preoperative antibiotics
  - Intraincisional antibiotics and antiseptics (controversial)
  - Peritoneal lavage
  - Surgical technique – speed, avoidance of spillage, isolation of infected organ using 'danger towel' technique

ANTISEPTICS USED[15]

- Alcohol (70% Isopropyl)
  - Bactericidal but evaporates and is short acting
  - Avoid in wounds since neuro toxic
- Halogens
  - Hypochlorite (Eusol, Milton's solution)
  - Iodoforms (iodine in alcohol)
    - Both are bactericidal and sporicidal and include *Staphylococcus*
    - Limited by patient hypersensitivity
- Quaternary ammonium (Cetrimide, Chlorhexidine)
  - Bactericidal not sporicidal
  - *Pseudomonas* can grow in it
- Dyes – Proflavine, Gentian violet – useful with Gram-positive cocci except *Staphylococcus* and no use in slough
- Formaldehyde (Noxythiolin) – releases 1% Formaldehyde and is useful in peritoneal lavage
- Silver sulphadiazine (Flamazine) – kills *Pseudomonas* and is useful in burns
- Phenols
  - Of historical interest (Lister)
  - Problems – absorption may lead to neurotoxicity
  - Staphylococcal resistance

ANTISEPTICS COMMONLY USED IN GENERAL SURGICAL PRACTICE[14]

Name	Presentation	Uses	Comments
Alcohol			
Alcohol	70% eythl, isopropyl	Skin preparation	
Quaternary ammonium			
Chlorhexidine (Hibiscrub)	Alcoholic 0.5% Aqueous 4%	Skin preparation Skin preparation. Surgical scrub. In dilute solutions in open wounds.	Has cumulative effect. Effective against Gram-positive organisms and relatively stable in the presence of pus and body fluids.
Cetrimide Aqueous (Savlon)		Handwashing. Instrument and surface cleaning	*Pseudomonas* spp. may grow in stored contaminated solutions. Ammonium compounds have a good detergent action (surface active agent)
Halogens			
Povidone-iodine (Betadine)	Alcoholic 10% Aqueous 7.5%	Skin preparation. Skin preparation. Surgical scrub. In dilute solution in open wounds	Safe, fast-acting broad spectrum. Some sporicidal sctivity. Antifungal. Iodine is not free but combined with polyvinylpyrrolidone (povidone). Should be reserved for use as disinfectant.
Hypochlorytes (Eusol, Milton, Chloramine T)	Aqueous preparations	Instrument and surface cleaning (debriding agent in open wounds?)	

PROPHYLACTIC USE OF ANTIBIOTICS

- Use for the shortest possible time commencing with premedication or induction
- If the course lasts for >24 h it should be considered therapeutic not prophylactic
- Choice of antibiotic depends on:
  - Suspected organism
  - Route of administration
  - Route of metabolism/excretion
  - Patient tolerance
  - Site of infection

THERAPEUTIC USE OF ANTIBIOTICS

When considering using an antibiotic for 'surgical' infection always consider:
- Is there pus to drain?
- Would lavage better?
- Is physiotherapy more appropriate?
- Is there another cause for the pyrexia, e.g. DVT

PROPHYLACTIC ANTIBIOTICS[10]

Clinical situation	Likely organism(s)	Prophylactic regimen
Appendicectomy	Anaerobes	Metronidazole (single dose PR 1 hr pre-op.)
Biliary tract surgery	Coliforms	Cephalosporin (i.v. immediately pre-op. and for 24 h post-op.)
Colorectal surgery	Coliforms	Metronidazole + cephalosporin or gentamicin (i.v. immediately pre-op. and anaerobes for up to 48 h post-op.)
GU surgery instrumentation	Coliforms	Gentamicin (single i.v. dose pre-procedure)
Open surgery		Cephalosporin (i.v. immediately pre-op. and for 24–48 h post-op.) or gentamicin (single i.v. dose immediately pre-op.)
Insertion of prosthetic joints	Staph. aureus Staph. epidermidis	Flucloxacillin (i.v. immediately pre-op. and 24–48 h post-op.)
Amputation of limb	C. perfringens	Penicillin (i.v. immediately pre-op. and for 24 h post-op.)
Vascular surgery with prosthetic graft	Staph. aureus Staph. epidermidis Coliforms	Cephalosporin (i.v. immediately pre-op. and for 24 h post-op.)
Prevention of tetanus in contaminated wound (+ immunoprophylaxis)	C. tetanus	Penicillin (i.v. or i.m. on presentation)
Prophylaxis of endocarditis		
Minor dental	Oral streptococci	Amoxycillin (single oral dose 1 h pre-op. Clindamycin if allergic)
Major dental		Low risk procedure – amoxycillin (oral dose 4 h pre-op. and one dose post-op.) High risk procedure – amoxycillin and gentamicin (i.m. or i.v. immediately pre-op. Vancomycin if allergic)
Genitorurinary instrumentation	Coliforms	Amoxycillin + gentamicin (i.v. immediately pre-op.)

All regimens are intravenous and should start preoperatively. In elective operations, antibiotics can be given at induction of anaesthesia. In emergency operations (or in contamination during elective surgery) antibiotics should be given at diagnosis and prolonged as therapy for 3–5 days if necessary.

WOUND INFECTION RATES CURRENTLY SEEN AFTER GENERAL SURGICAL OPERATIONS[14]

Type of surgery	Infection rate	Rate before prophylaxis
Clean (no viscus opened)	1–2%	The same
Clean-contaminated (viscus opened, minimal spillage)	<10%	Gastric surgery up to 30% Biliary surgery up to 20%
Contaminated (open viscus with spillage or inflammatory disease)	15–20%	Variable but up to 60%
Dirty (pus or perforation, incision through an abscess)	<40%	Up to 60% or more

THE IDEAL SURGICAL DRESSING[14]

- Is absorbent and can remove excess exudate
- Maintains a moist environment and aids tissues to debride necrotic material and promotes healing
- Prevents trauma to the underlying healing granulation tissue, or prevents the shedding of foreign particles into the wound
- Is leak proof and prevents strike-through and secondary infection
- Maintains temperature and gaseous change
- Allows simple dressing changes, easy, less frequent applications and removal, and is pain-free
- Is odourless, cosmetically acceptable and comfortable
- Is inexpensive

TYPES OF SURGICAL DRESSINGS[14]

Type	Name (example)	Indications and comments
Debriding agents	Benoxyl-benzoic and salacylic acid Aserbine-benzoic and salacylic acid Variclene-lactic acid	Used only in necrotic sloughing skin ulcers. Provide acidic environment. Claimed to enhance healing with debriding action.
Enzymatic agents	Varidase-streptokinase/ streptodornase	Activate fibrinolysis and liquify pus on chronic skin ulcers.
Bead dressings	Debrisan Iodosorb Other paste dressings	Remove bacteria and excess moisture by capillary action in deep granulating wounds. Antimicrobials may be added but with questionable topical benefit.
Polymeric films	Opsite Bioclusive Tegaderm	Primary adhesive transparent dressing for sutured wounds or donor sites.
Foams	Silastic (elastomer) Lyofoam Allevyn	Elastomeric dressing can be shaped to fit deep cavities and granulating wounds. Absorbent and non-adherent.
Hydrogels	Geliperm Intrasite	Maintain moist environment. Polymers can absorb exudate, or antiseptics (but adding antiseptics is of doubtful benefit). Semipermeable but allow gas exchange.
Hydrocolloids	Cornfeel Granuflex	Complete occlusion. Promote epithelialisation and granulation tissue. Maintain moisture without gaseous exchange across them.
Fibrous polymers	Kaltostat Sorbsan	Absorptive alginate dressings. Derived from natural (seaweed) source. Like polymeric hydrocolloids and hydrogels can pack deep wounds.

Type	Name (example)	Indications and comments
Biological membranes Simple miscellaneous	Porcine skin, amnion	Used for superficial chronic skin ulcers. No proven advantage.
	Gauzes: viscose/cotton with nonadherent coating (Melolin) Tulles: nonadherent paraffin impregnation	Simple absorptive dressing used only as a secondary dressing to absorb exudate. Added microbials probably confer no benefit. Added charcoal absorbents may reduce swelling. Relatively cheap but of questionable effectiveness.

VENOUS THROMBOEMBOLIC DISEASE

DEEP VEIN THROMBOSIS (DVT)[15]

Incidence (percentages includes subclinical cases using labelled fibrinogen)

- Major surgery 40%
  - Aetiology – Virchow's triad
  - Blood hypercoagubility
  - Vessel wall damage
  - Decreased flow
  - Increased viscosity
- Multiple injuries 60%
  - Aetiology – Virchow's triad
  - Antithrombin III, lupus anticoagulant, heparin cofactor, protein C, protein S, a-I antitrypsin, fibrinolytic impairment, oral contraceptive, smoking increases plasma fibrinogen
  - Increased packed cell volume
  - Stasis during surgery or bed rest
  - Compression, trauma, radiotherapy

FACTORS INCREASING THE RISK OF DEEP VEIN THROMBOSIS[14]

- Patient factors
- Age
- Obesity
- Varicose veins
- Immobility (bed rest over 4 days)
- Pregnancy
- Puerperium
- High dose oestrogen therapy
- Previous deep vein
- Thrombosis or pulmonary embolism
- Thrombophilia
- Deficiency of anti-thrombin III, protein C or protein S
- Antiphospholipid antibody or lupus anticoagulant

- Disease or surgical procedures
- Trauma or surgery, especially of pelvis, hip, lower limb
- Malignancy, especially pelvic, abdominal, metastatic

- Heart failure
- Recent myocardial infection
- Paralysis of the lower limb(s)
- Infection
- Inflammatory bowel disease
- Nephrotic syndrome
- Polycythaemia
- Paraproteinaemia
- Paroxysmal nocturnal haemoglobinuria
- Behçet's disease
- Homocystinaemia

RISK PREDICTION[14]

	Deep vein thrombosis	Proximal vein thrombosis	Fatal pulmonary embolism	Recommended prophylaxis
Low risk groups	<10%	<1%	0.01%	Graduated compression stocking with early ambulation

- Minor surgery (<30 min); no risk factors other than age
- Major surgery (>30 min); age <40 years or other risk factors*
- Minor trauma or medical illness

Moderate risk groups	10–40%	1–10%	0.1–1%	Low dose heparin or EPC*

- Major general, urological, gynaecological, cardiothoracic, vascular or neurological surgery; age >40: no other risk factor
- Major medical illness: heart or lung disease, cancer, inflammatroy bowel disease
- Major trauma or burns
- Minor surgery, trauma or illness in patients with previous DVT, pulmonary embolism (PE) or thrombophilia
- >40 years and operations > 30 min

High risk groups	40–80%	10–30%	1–10%	Combined regimens or i.v. heparin

- Fracture or major orthopaedic surgery of pelvis, hip or lower limb
- Major pelvic or abdominal surgery for malignant disease
- Major surgery, trauma or illness in patients with previous DVT, PE or thrombophilia
- Lower limb paralysis (e.g. hemiplegic stroke, paraplegia)
- Major lower limb amputations
- Recent venous thrombo-embolism, extensive additional surgery

DIAGNOSIS OF DVT[8,15]

- History and examination
- Swollen painful calf and leg
- Pulmonary embolism
- Positive Homan's sign unreliable
- Doppler calf studies

---

* EPC = external pneumatic compression

- Plethsmography
- Venography
- Isotope labelled fibrinogen/streptokinase

DVT PROPHYLAXIS[8,15]

- Mechanical
  - Compression stockings (TED)
  - Pulsion pneumatic compression
  - Electrical calf muscle stimulation
  - Foot pedals
  - Ankle rests to elevate calves
- Pharmacological
  - 'Mini dose' heparin, 5000 units b.d. (premed until full mobilization) reduces the incidence of DVT from 40 to 10%
  - Dextran 70 infusion for 2 days reduces platelet adhesivness reduces incidence from 40 to 20%
  - Warfarin
  - Note: aspirin is not proven to reduce DVT
- Postoperative care
  - Early mobilization
  - Avoid calf compression and leg crossing
  - Good hydration
  - Graduated compression stockings

TREATMENT OF DVT[15]

- Anticoagulation – fully heparinize, checking thrombin time, then warfarinize for 6 months checking prothrombin time regularly
- Streptokinase – if the thrombus is large, it is likely to embolize, has not occurred in the immediate postoperative period or in a patient with a history of peptic ulceration
- Thrombectomy – if venogram suggests that it is not fixed
- IVC plication filter

DIAGNOSIS AND TREATMENT OF PULMONARY EMBOLISM[15]

- Accounts for 5% of hospital deaths
- Usually occurs 7–12 days post-surgery
- Is associated with iliofemoral and pelvic DVT (note: only 30% of patients have clinically proven DVT)
- Diagnosis
  - History and examination
    - Dyspnoea
    - Pleuritic chest pain
    - Haemoptysis
    - Atelectasis
    - Increased JVP, elevated CVP

- – Decreased cardiac output
- – Cardiopulmonary collapse
- Special investigations
  - Chest X-ray
    - – Wedge-shaped collapse
    - – Pleural effusion on chest X-ray
    - – ECG S1 Q3 T wave inversion – right heart strain on chest leads
  - Blood gas – hypoxia
  - Ventilation perfusion scan – ventilation and perfusion mismatch (ventilation normal, perfusion deficient)
  - Baseline clotting prior to anticoagulation (pulmonary angiography, increased LDH)
- Treatment
  - Medical
    - Anticoagulate as for DVT
    - Streptokinase
  - Surgical
    - Trendelenberg pulmonary embolectomy
    - Caval interruption; plication/filter

FAT EMBOLISM[29]

Aetiology (two theories)
- Mechanical – bone marrow enters the blood stream through torn venous channels
- Metabolic – chylomicrons aggregate as secondary effect of trauma due to release of lipases from damaged tissue

Signs of fat embolism
- Unexplained pyrexia (usually 12–24 h after injury) too early to be infective
- Altered consciousness due to cerebral oedema and microinfarcts
- Tachycardia
- Raised or normal respiratory rate
- Hypercapnia
- Hypoxia (PO_2 usually [ss]8 kPa)
- Skin petechiae of the trunk and limbs
- Clotting abnormalities vary from mild to disseminated intravascular coagulation (thrombocytopenia due to formation of pulmonary aggregates)

Treatment
- High-flow oxygen therapy. Ventilation if the PO_2 cannot be maintained >8 kPa
- PEEP can reopen collapsed alveoli. Neither heparin nor corticosteroids have been proven to be of benefit

Prognosis
- The fully established syndrome is associated with a mortality rate of 10–15%

ANASTOMOSES

SITES OF COMMON ANASTOMOSES[14]

Gastrointestinal	Urological	Vascular
Oesophagus	Ureter	Aorta
Stomach	Bladder	Peripheral artery (e.g. femoral)
Small intestine	Urethra	Vein (e.g. portal)
Biliary or pancreatic	Vas deferens	Lymphatic
Large intestine		Coronary artery
		Microvascular (e.g. cerebral)

FACTORS INFLUENCING ANASTOMOTIC HEALING

General	Specific	Local
Age (e.g. infancy and old age)	Anaemia	Site of anastomosis
Circumstances	Suture line disease	Oesophagus
Elective surgery	Irradiated tissue	Rectum
Emergency surgery	Infected anastomosis	Extra peritoneal
Obstructed bowel	Antibiotics	Proximal faecal loading
Malignancy		Dilated proximal bowel
Sepsis		Suture technique
Drugs		Mucosal inversion
Corticosteroids		One v. two layer
Immunosuppressives		Suture material
Malnutrition		Absorbent v.
		non-absorbent
Anaemia		Good blood supply
Jaundice		No tension
Uraemia		Drain
Irradiation		Stimuli (e.g. feeding or drugs)

FISTULAE

CAUSES OF A PERSISTENCE OF A SINUS OR FISTULA[14]

- A foreign body or necrotic tissue is present, e.g. a suture, hairs, a sequestrum, a faecolith or even a (Guinea) worm.
- Inefficient or non-dependent drainage. A long, narrow, tortuous track predisposes to inefficient drainage.
- Unrelieved obstruction of the lumen of a viscus or tube distal to the fistula.
- Absence of rest, such as occurs in fistula-in-ano due to the normal contractions of the sphincter which also forces faecal material into the internal opening.

- Walls have become lined with epithelium or endothelium (arteriovenous fistula).
- Dense fibrosis prevents contraction and healing.
- Type of infection, e.g. tuberculosis or actinomycosis.
- Presence of malignant disease.
- Persistent discharge such as urine, faeces or cerebrospinal fluid.
- Ischaemia.
- Drugs, e.g. steroids.
- Malnutrition.
- Interference, e.g. artefacts irradiation, e.g. recto-vaginal fistula after treatment for a carcinoma of the cervix.
- Treatment – remedy depends on the removal or the specific treatment of the cause (see page 121).

COMMON OPERATIVE INJURIES[5]

Organ	Operation/procedure	Risk factors
Oesophagus	Para-oesophageal surgery; fundoplication, vagotomy, repair hiatus hernia	Oesophagitis, previous surgery
Spleen	Para-oesophageal and gastric surgery	Splenomegaly, perisplenitis, mobilisation of splenic flexure
Pancreas	Splenectomy	Bleeding from the mobilised spleen or hilar vessels
Bile duct	Cholecystectomy	Abnormal anatomy, inadequate display, omission of operative cholangiography, difficult cholecystectomy, bleeding
Duodenum	Right hemicolectomy	Adhesion of hepatic flexure to third part of duodenum
Small intestine	Enterolysis	Dilated, oedematous intestinal loops
Ureter	Hysterectomy, colectomy	Inadequate identification of ureter, devascularisation, involvement of inflammatory mass

Note: operative injuries to the spleen account for 16–20% of all splenectomies. Injury to the abdominal oesophagus occurs in 0.9% of all vagotomies.

3

SURGICAL SUPPORT

INTENSIVE CARE UNIT (ICU)

- 1:1 nursing care
- 1:4/5 dedicated clinician
- Mechanical ventilatory support
- Advanced close monitoring support

INDICATIONS FOR ADMISSION

- Support and control of vital organ function
  - Respiratory – mechanical ventilation
  - Renal – haemofiltration
  - Cardiac – ECG, inotropic drugs
  - Hepatic – transfusion of blood products
- Monitoring of unstable patients
  - Oxygenation – RR, saturation, PO_2/ PCO_2/ pH
  - Cardiac/renal function – pulse, BP, CVP, pulmonary wedge pressure
  - Cardiac output/systemic vascular resistance – urine output
  - Haematology/biochemistry
- Problems requiring close nursing attention not possible on general ward (wound care, drains / lines, unstable patient)

SURGICAL ADJUNCTS

DIATHERMY

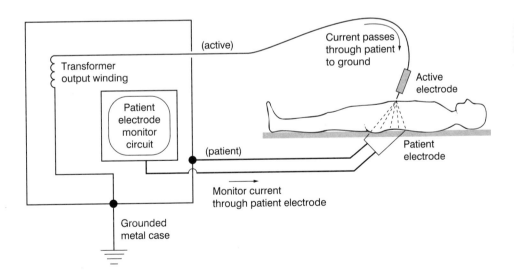

Figure 3.1 Components of a standard monopolar diathermy circuit using the correct earthing system and application of the indifferent (patient's electrode).

Key features
- Passage of alternating current at high frequency through body tissue
- Local concentration produces heat
- Frequency range 400 KHz to 10 MHz, current up to 500 mA for safe use
- Heat up to 1000°C
  - Cutting tissue effect – continuous output
  - Coagulation effect – pulsed output

Monopolar
- Current pathway through body via plate
- Maximal current density at point of smallest cross-sectional area
- Not for use on extremities (penis)

Bipolar
- Current passes through tissue between forcep points
- Lower current, safer

Risks

- Burns
  - Capacitance coupling
  - Inadvertent/excess use of probe
  - Poor positioning of earthing plate
  - Use of monopolar on appendages
  - Explosions if used near volatile gas
- Pacemakers – may interfere with rhythm

LASERS

LASER = **L**ight **A**mplification by the **S**timulated **E**mission of **R**adiation

Types of lasers in medical use
- Carbon dioxide
  - Rapid absorption > minimal penetration
  - Excision of skin blemishes, tattoos
  - Haemostasis in ENT surgery
  - Premalignant cervical/vulval lesions
- Nd-YAG (neodymium-yttrium aluminium garnet)
  - 3–5 mm penetration
  - Coagulation effect, causes scarring
  - Destruction of tumours, e.g. oesophagus palliation, duodenum, rectal tumours, bladder tumours
  - Haemostasis in GI bleeding, liver bed, ulcers
  - Laser angioplasty in vascular surgery
  - Posterior capsule destruction in cataract surgery
- Argon
  - Absorbed by red pigment
  - Retinal detachment, trabeculoplasty
  - Skin blemishes

Risks

- Patient
  - Excessive burning
  - Scar formation
  - Perforation of viscus
  - Damage to surrounding tissues
- Operator – accidental exposure over skin/eyes – corneal burns/cataract

CARDIOPULMONARY BYPASS

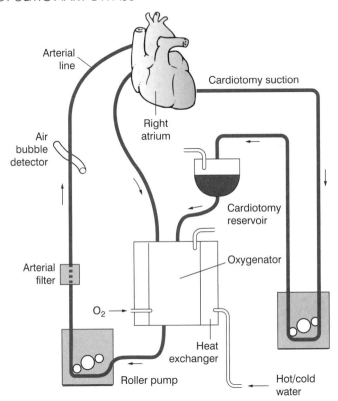

Figure 3.2 Components of a standard cardiopulmonary bypass circuit.

MINIMALLY INVASIVE SURGERY

Types of minimally invasive surgery[14]

- Laparoscopic operations
  - Cholecystostomy
  - Cholecystectomy
  - Common duct exploration
  - Cholecystojejunostomy for malignant jaundice
  - Deroofing of hepatic cysts
  - Appendicectomy

- Femoral/inguinal hernia repair
- Cardiomyotomy
- Ligamentum teres cardiopexy
- Partial (Toupet, Dor) fundoplication
- Crural repair and total fundoplication
- Suture toilet of perforated duodenal ulcer
- Vagotomy: truncal, HSV (highly selective vagotomy), others
- Varicocele
- Rectopexy
- Nephrectomy
- Thorascopic operations
  - Thoracodorsal sympathectomy
  - Ligature of bullae and pleurectomy/pleurodesis
  - Pulmonary wedge lobar, total resections
  - Pericardiectomy
  - Long oesophageal myotomy
  - Oesophagectomy
- Combined approaches
  - Endoscopic – open access
    - Right hemicolectomy
    - Left hemicolectomy
  - Combined endoscopic – oesophagogastectomy with cervical anastomosis
  - Endoscopic – left colectomy

Benefits and risks of laparoscopic surgery (see pages 82–83)

SURGICAL PHARMACOLOGY

DRUG-INDUCED GASTROINTESTINAL AND HEPATOBILIARY DISORDERS[5]

Disorder	Drug
Ulcers and haemorrhages	Aspirin and NSAIDs
Strictures	Potassium chloride
Pseudo-obstruction	Tricyclic antidepressants, MAOI, narcotic analgesics, excess purgation
Cholestatic jaundice and hepatitis	Adverse drug reactions
Peliosis hepatitis	Androgens, oestrogens, methotrexate
Focal nodular hyperplasia	Oral contraceptives, androgens and hepatic adenomas
Hepatocellular carcinomas	Androgens, oral contraceptives
Reye's syndrome	Aspirin in children
Acute cholecystitis	Diuretics, ?parenteral nutrition

DRUG-INDUCED ENDOCRINE AND METABOLIC DISORDERS

Disorder	Drug
Hyperprolactinaemia	Phenothiazines, benzodiazepines, monoamine oxidase inhibitors, metoclopramide, butyrophenones
Growth retardation	Corticosteroids, androgens
Hyperthyroidism	Iodide preparations, amiodarone, lithium
Hypothyroidism	Sulphonylureas, phenylbutazone, aminoglutethimide, amiodarone, pentazocine, cyclophosphamide, ethionamide, lithium
Adrenal insufficiency	Steroids, metyrapone, aminoglutethimide, trilostane, ketoconazole, etomidate, oral anticoagulants
Gonadal dysfunction	Combination chemotherapy
Gynaecomastia	Oestrogens, spironolactone, digitalis, cimetidine, soniazid, ethionamide, griseofulvin
Dilutional hyponatraemia	Chlorpropamide, carbamazepine, vincristine, cyclophosphamide, cisplatin
Partial nephrogenic diabetes insipidus	Lithium, demeclocycline
Osteoporosis	Steroids

DRUG-INDUCED GENITO-URINARY DISORDERS

Disorder	Drug
Papillary necrosis	Phenacetin, amidopyrine, etc.
Renal failure	Neomycin, cephaloridine, cephalin, colistin, vancomycin, amphotericin, cisplatin, penicillamine, cyclosporin, anti-inflammatory drugs, etc.
Retention of urine	Anticholinergic drugs, narcotic analgesics, diuretics
Epididymitis	Amiodarone

DRUG-INDUCED HAEMATOLOGICAL DISORDERS

Disorder	Drug
Myelosuppression	Cytotoxic agents, carbimazole, sulphonamides, etc.
Bleeding tendency (potentiation of warfarin)	NSAIDs, co-trimoxazole, metronidazole, latamoxef, cephamandole, erythromycin, neomycin, ketoconazole, miconazole, alcohol, danazol, clofibrate, cimetidine, anabolic steroids, etc.
Haemolysis	Salazopyrine, sulphonamides, aspirin, etc.
Thrombosis	Oral contraceptives

DRUG-INDUCED NEUROMUSCULAR DISORDERS

Disorder	Drug
Postoperative respiratory depression	Aminoglycosides, polymyxins, tetracyclines, lincomycin, clindamycin, chloroquine
Suxamethonium apnoea	Phenelzine, ecothiopate, aprotinin, ketamine, procaine, promazine, lignocaine, clindamycin, lincomycin, lithium
Aggravation of myasthenia gravis	Aminoglycosides, procainamide, β-blockers, chloroquine, phenytoin, lithium, etc.
Myasthenic syndrome	Aminoglycosides, polymyxins, anticonvulsants, β-blockers

DRUG-INDUCED PSYCHIATRIC DISORDERS

Disorder	Drug
Delirium	Hypnotics, alcohol, most anti-depressants, neuroleptics, anti-histamines, hyoscine, atropine, β-blockers, digoxin, cimetidine
Psychotic states	Phenylephrine, salbutamol, propranolol, levodopa, bromocriptine, pentazocine, dihydro-codeine, indomethacin
Mania	Tricyclics, MAOIs, corticosteroids, aminophylline, levodopa
Depression	Methyldopa, clonidine, propanolol, phenobarbitone, corticosteroids, indomethacin, fenfluramine, oral contraceptives, chloroquine, cycloserine

DRUGS TO BE AVOIDED IN PREGNANCY[14]

In early pregnancy – potentially teratogenic	In later pregnancy – foetal and perinatal effects	Use with particular caution
Cytotoxic drugs	Sex steroids	All CNS depressants
Sex steroids	Warfarin	Lithium
Retinoids	Tetracyclines	Antithyroid drugs
Warfarin	Sulphonamides	Corticosteroids
Anticonvulsants*	Chloramphenicol	
Tetracyclines	Alcohol	
	Tobacco	
	Non-steroidal anti-inflammatory drugs	
	Sulphonylureas	

* Some controversy but probably all are teratogenic. Sodium valproate may be most hazardous. However, the danger of drugs must be weighed against the danger of uncontrolled seizures.

DRUGS THAT SHOULD BE AVOIDED IN SEVERE RENAL FAILURE (GLOMERULAR FILTRATION RATE <10 ml/min)[14]

Aspirin	Platelet dysfunction, gastrointestinal symptoms
Tetracyclines	Deterioration of renal function (except doxycycline, minocycline)
Nalidixic acid	Systemic lupus erythematosus-like syndrome due to metabolites
Nitrofurantoin	Peripheral neuropathy
Methotrexate	Nephrotoxic
Amiloride	Hyperkalaemia, acidosis
Thiazides	Ineffective, hyperuricaemia
Spironolactone	Hyperkalaemia, acidosis
Probenecid	Ineffective, possible uric acid stones
Chlorpropamide	Hypoglycaemia
Gallamine	Prolonged apnoea
Pancuronium	Prolonged apnoea
Penicillamine	Nephrotic syndrome
Aurothiomalate sodium	Nephrotoxic

4

SURGICAL ONCOLOGY

COMMON MALIGNANCIES

Tumour site	Approximate number of deaths p.a.
Bronchus/lung	35,000
Breast	14,000
Colon/rectum	16,000
Prostate	12,000
Stomach	9000
Pancreas	6000
Oesophagus	5000
Lymphoma	9000
Total in UK	150,000

PATHOPHYSIOLOGICAL FACTORS

- Genetic – specific chromosome locations
- Environmental
  - Radiation exposure
  - Industrial toxins/irritants
  - Dietary factors

SYMPTOMS AND SIGNS

- Local
  - Swelling, inflammation, pain
  - Obstruction – venous, visceral (bowel, biliary system, bladder, CNS)
  - Bleeding
  - Invasion, perforation
- Distant
  - Cachexia
  - Ascites
  - Pleural effusion

STAGING

Systems based on tumour progression

- Local – **T**umour size, invasion
- Lymph **N**odes – local, distant
- **M**etastasis

PRINCIPLES OF MANAGEMENT

Curative
- Removal of primary lesion
  - Complete surgical resection or ablation with normal tissue margins
  - Adjuvant treatment to remove possible residual disease
- Return to premorbid risk status

Palliative
- Non- or incomplete removal of primary lesion
  - Relief of obstruction
  - Debulking
- Presence of distant disease
  - Lymph nodes
  - Other organs
- Symptomatic treatment
  - Pain
  - Nausea
  - Cachexia
  - Social

ADJUVANT TREATMENT

- Hormonal
- Radiotherapy
- Chemotherapy

RADIOTHERAPY

Curative
- Results equivalent to or better than surgery
- Squamous cell carcinoma
  - Oesophagus
  - Skin
  - Cervix
  - Tongue/head and neck

Adjuvant
- Breast
- Colorectal
- CNS

Palliative
- Inaccessible/inoperable lesions
  - Metastatic deposits
  - Bone pain/collapse
  - Spinal cord compression
  - Superior vena caval obstruction

Radioresistant tumours
- Kidney
- Adenocarcinoma of stomach
- Malignant melanoma

PRINCIPLES

- Destruction of mitotic cells
- Normal cells also damaged
- Unit of absorbed radiation: 1 Gy = 1 J/kg

APPLICATION

- Implants
  - Iridium for carcinoma of tongue
  - Caesium for carcinoma of cervi
- External beam radiation – single large dose or multiple small doses (fractionation)
- Systemic radiation – [131]iodine for thyroid disease

COMPLICATIONS

- Skin
  - Burns
  - Ulceration/bleeding
- Lymphoedema
- Gastrointestinal tract
  - Mucositis
  - Oesophagitis
  - Enteritis
    - Bleeding
    - Diarrhoea
  - Stricture formation
- Gonadal damage
- Hypothyroidism
- Renal tubular damage
- Haematuria
- Fibrotic bladder
- Myocardial damage
- Late malignancies – acute leukaemia post-irradiation for Hodgkin's

CHEMOTHERAPY

ADVANCED TUMOURS WHICH ARE POTENTIALLY CURABLE[14]

- Acute lymphoblastic leukaemia
- Germ cell tumours
- Choriocarcinoma
- Ewing's sarcoma
- Hodgkin's disease
- Wilms' tumour
- Diffuse cell lung cancer
- ?Small cell lung cancer
- ?Ovarian cancer

TUMOURS THAT ARE POTENTIALLY CURABLE BY LOCAL TREATMENT AND ADJUVANT CHEMOTHERAPY[14]

- Breast cancer
- Osteogenic sarcoma

TUMOURS THAT HAVE A RESPONSE RATE WHICH LEADS TO PROLONGED SURVIVAL[14]

- Ovarian cancer
- Lymphoma
- Osteogenic sarcoma
- Breast cancer
- Acute myeloid leukaemia

TUMOURS THAT HAVE AN OVERALL RESPONSE RATE OF 50% BUT NO DEFINITE SURVIVAL BENEFIT[14]

- Head and neck cancer
- Bladder cancer
- Cervical cancer

TUMOURS THAT ARE POORLY RESPONSIVE TO CHEMOTHERAPY[14]

- Pancreatic cancer
- Melanoma
- Soft tissue sarcoma
- Colorectal cancer
- Renal cancer
- Thyroid cancer
- Gastric cancer
- Non-small cell lung cancer

PRINCIPLE

- Relative destruction of tumour cells with sparing of normal cells

DESTRUCTION OF MICRO-METASTATIC CELLS

Phase-dependent
- Kill cells with increasing dose, not dependant on cell cycle phase
  - Methotrexate
  - Procarbazine
  - Vinca alkaloids
  - Etoposide

Non-phase-dependent
- Kill cells at specific point in cycle, plateau at high doses
  - 5-Fluoruracil
  - Actinomycin D
  - Alkylating agents

COMPLICATIONS

- Application method
  - Central line/Hickmann line complications
  - Tissue damage due to extravasation
- Bone marrow suppression
- Gastrointestinal toxicity

- Nausea
- Vomiting
- Mucositis
- Diarrhoea
- Constipation
- Alopecia
- Conjunctivitis
- Cystitis
- Pulmonary fibrosis
- Cardiomyopathy
- Renal and hepatic impairment
- Late malignancy – acute leukaemia
- Gonadal damage

SCREENING FOR MALIGNANT DISEASE

Aim: screening a population for a disease before it naturally presents may serve to establish early diagnosis of a less advanced lesion with the scope for better curative treatment and, hence, overall survival benefit for the screened population.

Proof of benefit: better survival in a screened population against a non-screened population. At present there is only a national screening programme established for breast cancer, though its results are being evaluated.

Case for screening other diseases argued in:

- Colorectal cancer
- Prostate cancer
- Cervical cancer
- Ovarian cancer
- Gastric cancer (national screening programme in Japan)

Non-malignant diseases

- Abdominal aortic aneurysm
- Intracranial aneurysm

Principles of a screening programme

Disease
- Relatively high incidence
- High mortality/morbidity rates if untreated/late diagnosis
- Diagnostic tests available
- Established and proven treatment mode available for disease
- Early treatment of diseases beneficial to long-term prognosis of the patient
- Resources available to cope with extra demand of further treatment and investigation

Patient
- At risk of developing disease
- Compliant

- Motivated to attend a screening programme
- Prepared to take the consequences of the findings
  - Asymptomatic serious disease requiring surgery and further treatment
  - Equivocal findings requiring further investigation

Screening method

- Cheap
- Widely available
- Low-risk procedure
- Minimally invasive
- High sensitivity (low false-negative rate)
- High specificity rate (high true-positive rate)

BREAST CANCER

- Common disease, high mortality rate
- Improved survival in early diagnosis with established treatment method

National screening programme

- Women 50–64 years of age invited to attend
- One-off mammogram taken
  - Normal findings – invited for follow-up in 5 years
  - Abnormal findings – referred to clinician

Problems

- Compliance varies with region
- Women <50 years of age not suitable for this test
- 95–97% sensitivity; false-negative women may be inappropriately cleared of disease
- 85% specificity; large numbers of equivocal lesions
  - Require further investigations, including open biopsy
  - New risks for patient, increased resources to cope with follow-up
- How to deal with extensive DCIS/LCIS
- Small radiation dose of mammogram
- The provisional results of screening programme are to be published

COLORECTAL CANCER

- Tests
  - Faecal occult blood – low sensitivity, low specificity
  - Serum CEA – low sensitivity
  - Colonoscopy/barium enema
    - >95% sensitivity and specificity
    - Expensive, invasive, potential risks (1/100 risk of colonoscopic perforation)
- No suitable test yet available to establish major screening programme

PROSTATE CANCER

- Tests
  - Serum PSA – low specificity (raised in benign disease)
  - Prostatic biopsy – expensive, invasive, potential risks

Prostate cancer has its highest incidence in men >65 years of age; debate is ongoing about whether screening will alter the population survival rate.

GASTRIC CANCER

- Large established screening programme in Japan where the incidence of disease high
- Test
  - Upper gastrointestinal endoscopy
    - High sensitivity and specificity
    - Invasive and expensive
- Relatively low UK incidence of disease argues for a screening programme

ABDOMINAL AORTIC ANEURYSM

- USS aorta – high sensitivity, specificity (>99%)
- Problem of small (<5 cm) asymptomatic aneurysms
- Present risks in treatment of disease may outweigh the potential benefits of early diagnosis

THORACIC MALIGNANCY[12A]

PRIMARY PULMONARY NEOPLASIA

- 95% malignant
- Lung cancer causes 40 000 deaths in UK per annum (most common malignancy).

Risk factors

Enviromental

- Tobacco smoke
- Other pollutants/toxins
- Radon
- Arsenic
- Ethers
- Nickel
- Asbestos

Genetic

Classification

Primary lesions

- Epithelial lesions
  - Small cell carcinoma
    - 25% all lung cancers
    - Middle-aged/elderly patients
    - Neuroendocrine properties, i.e. can secrete neuropeptide hormones, ADH, ACTH, 5-HT, calcitonin (paraneoplastic syndromes)
    - Rapidly progressive, median survival 3 months
  - Squamous cell carcinoma
    - 40% lung cancers

- Elderly patients (over 60)
- Can secrete PTH or ACTH
  - Adenocarcinoma
    - 30% lung cancers
    - More common in women
    - Peripheral lesions
  - Large cell carcinoma
    - 10% lung cancers
- Rare
  - Adenosquamous carcinoma
  - Carcinoid tumours
  - Bronchial gland tumours
  - Sarcoma
  - Lymphoma
- Benign
  - Hamartoma
  - Chondroma
  - Granular cell tumour

Clinical features

General

- Cough
- Haemoptysis
- Wheezing
- Dyspnoea
- Recurrent pneumonia

Local invasions

- Recurrent laryngeal nerve   Voice change
- Phrenic nerve   Hemidiaphragmatic paresis
- Chest wall   Pain
- Superior vena cava   Dilated upper body / neck
- Oesophagus   Dysphagia
- Pericardium   Dysrhythmia

Paraneoplastic syndromes

- Hormonal
  - Cushings (ACTH)
  - Inappropriate anti-diuresis
  - Hypercalcaemia (Calcitonin)
  - Hypermetabolism (GH, TSH)
  - Gynaecomastia
- Constitutional effects
  - Anorexia
  - Cachexia
  - Hypertrophic pulmonary osteoarthropathy (clubbing)
- Dermatological
  - Browens disease
  - Erythema
  - Hypertrichosis

- Neuromuscular
  - Dermatomyositis
  - Polymyositis
  - Eaton-Lambert syndrome
- Neurological
  - Dementia
  - Peripheral neuropathy
- Haematological
  - Haemolytic anaemia
  - Disseminated intravascular coagulation

Investigations

- Chest X-ray
  - High sensitivity
  - 7% of lung cancer show calcification
- CT scan
  - Identifies intrathoracic/extrathoracic spread
- Sputum cytology
- Bronchoscopy and biopsy

Staging

TNM classification	
TIS	Carcinoma in situ
T1	<3 cm diameter, within visceral pleura, no invasion of local bronchus
T2	>3 cm diameter, or visceral pleural invasion, or bronchial obstruction to hilar region
T3	Invasion of chest wall, diaphragm, pericardium or mediastinal pleura, or lesions within 2 cm of carina
T4	Invasion of mediastinal structures, malignant pleural effusion
N0	No involved nodes
N1	Ipsilateral hilar or peribronchial nodes
N2	Ipsilateral mediastinal and/or subcarinal nodes
N3	Contralateral nodes, or ipsilateral supraclavicular/scalene nodes
M0	No disseminated disease
M1	Disseminated disease

Subclassification and prognosis		5 year survival
Stage I	Localised tumour, no nodes (T1–2, N0, M0)	80%
Stage II	Localised tumour, local nodes only (T1–2, N1, M0)	50%
Stage IIIa	Surgically resectable (T1–3, N1–2, M0)	20%
Stage IIIb	Non-resectable (T1–4, N1–3, M0)	5%
Stage IV	Metastatic disease (M1)	<5%

Management

- Surgical resection for early lesions ($\leqslant$T2) dependant on general condition of patient
- Adjuvant radiotherapy/chemotherapy
- Palliative treatment

TUMOUR MARKERS[21]

- A tumour marker is any substance related to the presence or progress of a tumour.
- Not all markers are tumour-specific.
- Markers may be secreted by tumours into the blood or serum (serum tumour markers), or expressed on the surface of tumour cells (tissue tumour markers).
- Tumour-derived markers are produced by the tumour. They may represent excessive secretion of a normal cellular product (e.g. calcitonin in thyroid medullary carcinoma or prostate-specific antigen [PSA] in prostate cancer) or the production of a substance not normally produced by the normal tissue (e.g. adrenocorticotrophic hormone in lung oat cell tumours).
- Tumour-associated markers are produced by non-malignant tumours cells as a result of the presence of a tumour (e.g. increased urinary hydroxyproline in skeletal metastases).

Tumour markers can be of value in:

1. Diagnosis
2. Screening
3. Estimation of tumour mass and staging
4. Tumour localization
5. Prognosis estimation
6. Prediction of response to or measurement after treatment
7. Detection of recurrences

SERUM TUMOUR MARKERS

Marker	Tumour	Uses (see previous list)
Prostate-specific antigen (PSA)	Prostatic carcinoma	1, ?2, 3, ?4, 5–7
β Human Chorionic Gonadotrophin (b-HCG)	Testicular teratoma	1–3, 5–7
α-Feto protein (AFP)	Testicular teratoma	1–3, 5–7
	Hepatoma	1, 6, 7
Carcinoembryonic antigen (CEA)	Colorectal carcinoma	3–7
Paraproteins	Myelomatosis	1, 3, 5–7
Eutopic hormones (normal hormones produced in excessive amounts from a normal site of origin, e.g.:		
Parathormone (PTH)	Parathyroid hormones	1, 4
ACTH	Cushing's disease	1, 4
GH	Pituitary adenoma	1
Calcitonin	Medullary thyroid carcinoma	1, 2, 6, 7

Insulin	Insulinoma	1, 2, 4, 6, 7
Catecholamines	Phaeochromocytoma	1, 2, 4
Gastrin	Gastrinoma	1–4, 6, 7
5-HT	Carcinoid tumour	1, 4, 6, 7
Erythropoietin	Renal cell carcinoma	6, 7

Ectopic hormones (an excess of hormone produced from abnormal sites)

ACTH	Bronchial and breast carcinoma	5, 6
ADH	Bronchial and breast carcinoma	5, 6
PTH	Bronchial and breast carcinoma	5, 6
Calcitonin	Bronchial and breast carcinoma	5, 6

Tissue tumour markers

Oestrogen receptors	Breast carcinoma	5, 6
Epithelial membrane antigen	Epithelial tumours	1
Carcinoembryonic antigen	Breast carcinoma	1
	Bronchial carcinoma	1
T cell, B cell markers	Lymphomas	1
	Leukaemias	1, 5
Common ALL antigen	Acute Lymphoblastic leukaemia	5, 6
HLe–1	Reticuloendothelial tumours	1

CHEMICALS AND FOODS RECOGNIZED AS CARCINOGENIC IN THE HUMAN[5]

Chemicals

- Carcinogen – target in the human
- 2-Naphthylamine
- Benzidine
- 4-Aminobiphenyl – urinary bladder
- 4-Nitrobiphenyl
- N,N-bis(2-chloroethyl)–2-naphthylamine
- Bis (2-chloroethyl) sulphide
- Chromium compounds – lungs
- Chloromethyl methyl ether
- Cigarette smoke – lungs, pancreas, other tissues
- Certain soots, tars, oils, arsenic compounds – lungs, skin
- Asbestos – lungs, pleura
- Nickel compounds – lungs, nasal tissue
- Betel nuts – buccal mucosa
- Vinyl chloride – liver
- Diethylstilboestrol – vagina

Food

- Carcinogen from green plants
  - Cycasin
  - Nitrosamines and nitrosamides

- Pyrrolizidine alkaloids
- Allyl and propenyl benzine derivatives
- Polycyclic hydrocarbons
- Carcinogen elaborated by fungi
  - Aflatoxins
  - Sterigmatocystin
  - Yellow rice toxins
  - Griseofulvin
- Carcinogens produced by actinomycetes and bacteria
  - *Streptomyces* products
  - Actinomycin D
  - Mitomycin C
  - Streptozocin
  - Ethionine
  - Nitrosamines
- Carcinogens from animal meat – fat
- Industrial carcinogens and pesticides

CANCERS ASSOCIATED WITH CLINICAL SYNDROMES[5]

Disease	Tumour susceptibility	Mode of transfer
Neurofibromatosis	Glioma, meningioma, phaeochromocytoma, sarcoma	Autosomal dominant
Tuberous sclerosis	Glioma, neurofibroma, astrocytoma, phaeochromocytoma	Autosomal dominant
Von Hippel–Lindau	Haemangioblastomas, renal cell carcinoma	Autosomal dominant
Porphyria cutaneous tarda	BCC, hepatocellular carcinoma	Autosomal dominant
Polyposis coli	Carcinoma colon	Autosomal dominant
Gardner's syndrome	Carcinoma colon, endocrine carcinoma	Autosomal dominant
Peutz–Jegher's syndrome	Ovarian, carcinoma duodenum, and small bowel	Autosomal dominant
Ataxia telangiectasia	Leukaemia, reticuloses	Autosomal recessive
Albinism	BCC, SCC	Autosomal recessive
Tyrosinaemia	Hepatocellular carcinoma	Autosomal recessive
IgA deficiency	Lymphoreticular also carcinoma stomach, bladder, breast	Not clear
IgM deficiency	Lymphoreticular, neuroblastoma	Not clear

PALLIATIVE CARE

Involves evaluation and treatment of physical, psychological. social (cultural) and spiritual aspects to improve overall quality of life (**Figures 4.1 and 4.2**).

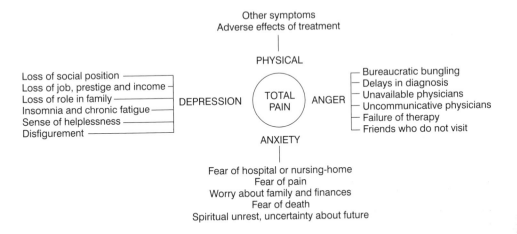

Figure 4.1 'Total pain' (as described by Twycross 1994).

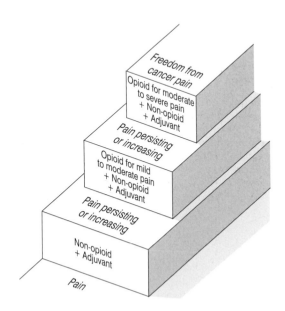

Figure 4.2 WHO 'ladder' for treatment of pain.

INDICATIONS FOR PALLIATIVE RADIOTHERAPY[5]

- Relief of pain
- Healing of ulceration
- Control of haemorrhage
- Relief of obstruction
- Suppression of effusions
- Relief of neurological symptoms
- Control of systemic symptoms and signs

5

GASTROINTESTINAL SYSTEM

ACUTE ABDOMEN

A clinical diagnosis indicating potentially serious intra-abdominal pathology that demands urgent management through resuscitation and probable surgical intervention.

PERITONITIS

An irritation or inflammation of the peritoneum resulting in clinical signs either localized to a specific area or generalized throughout the abdomen.

Causes
- Pus, bowel contents (upper – bilious/lower – faeculent), blood, necrotic debris

SURGICAL ACUTE ABDOMEN

Requiring immediate or delayed intervention:

Upper gastrointestinal
- Oesophageal, gastric or duodenal perforation

Hepatobiliary
- Cholecystitis
- Rupture gallbladder
- Ruptured liver or spleen

Lower gastrointestinal
- Appendicitis
- Inflamed Meckel's
- Inflammatory bowel disease causing obstruction, perforation, severe exacerbation or megacolon
- Neoplasia causing obstruction or perforation
- Diverticulitis (complications of)
- Ischaemic bowel
- Incarcerated hernia causing ischaemia/obstruction

Retroperitoneum
- Pancreatitis
- Ruptured abdominal aortic aneurysm
- Ureteric obstruction (renal colic)

Pelvic
- Rupture or torsion ovarian cyst
- Torsion testicle

Diagnosis

History
- Abdominal pain
  - Specific characteristics and natural history
  - Local or generalized
- Anorexia, nausea, vomiting

- Change in bowel habit – sudden or gradual onset
- Micturition – frequency, dysuria
- Fevers, chills, rigors

Examination

- Temperature, pulse, BP, RR (UO)
- Other systems
- General (nutrition, jaundice, anaemia, etc.)

Investigations

- FBC, U&E, amylase
  - ABG
  - LFTs, Ca, bone
- CXR (erect), AXR (supine)
- ECG
- Urinalysis/pregnancy test
- Specific to diagnosis (if available and indicated)

Resuscitation

- Oxygen
- i.v. access – fluid rehydration
- Central access
- NBM, nasogastric tube
- Catheterization
- Monitoring T, p, RR, BP, UO, CVP

Surgery

- Laparotomy/specific to presumed diagnosis
- Midline – most
- Gridiron-appendicitis
- Transverser Kockers – cholecystitis

Causes of abdominal pain that are often forgotten[12]

- Pancreatitis
- Aneurysm (leaking or dissecting)
- Mesenteric ischaemia
- Tabes dorsalis
- Epididymo orchitis
- Gynaecological (ovarian cyst, PID, ectopic pregnancy – see below)

Medical causes of acute abdominal pain[5]

- Myocardial infarction – the epigastrium is the sole site of the pain in 0.7% of cases and it occurs at any time in 3.3%. May be misdiagnosed as peptic ulceration.
- Lobar pneumonia – pain may be referred to either the subcostal region depending on the site of the lung disease. It is a problem often encountered in the elderly.
- Diabetic ketoacidosis – may present with abdominal pain and vomiting. A diabetic history may not be obtained particularly in the young juvenile previously undiagnosed diabetic. Urine testing for sugar and ketones should be performed on all patients admitted with acute abdominal pain.
- Acute hepatitis – viral or acute alcoholic hepatitis. Abdominal pain and tenderness is often present. The latter may be marked. The associated fever and jaundice may be

misinterpreted as cholangitis due to ductal calculi. The diagnosis should become clear by the marked elevation in the serum transaminases. Often, the level of consciousness is impaired.

- Sickle cell disease – the crises of this disorder, which are precipitated by hypoxia, produce both abdominal pain and tenderness.
- Henoch–Schonlein purpura – may present with acute colicky abdominal pain, nausea and vomiting usually in children and young adults with a preponderance in males. Intestinal infarction and perforation may occur in this condition which is due to the deposition of IgA–immune complexes.
- Congenital spherocytosis – abdominal pain is caused by acute haemolytic episodes
- Congenital erythropoietic – abdominal pain, vomiting and constipation. The erythropoietic type is precipitated by drugs, menstruation, hepatic porphyrias starvation, infection and alcohol excess.
- Acute porphyria – abdominal pain sometimes jaundice simulating common bile duct obstruction. Note: protoporphyrin can only be excreted in the bile. Attacks precipitated by fasting, sun exposure or iron deficiency.
- Herpes zoster – the pain most commonly in the distribution of the T7–L1 may precede blisters. The pain is of a burning nature and is usually quite severe.
- Lead poisoning – may present with episodes of intestinal colic. A blue line may be present in the gums.
- Campylobacter infections – these may cause pseudoappendicitis syndrome, acute terminal ileitis and mesenteric lymphadenitis. However, some of these infections may cause perforation and peritonitis.

Note: porphyrias are inherited disorders of porphyrin (haem precursor) metabolism. The main abnormalities occur either in the bone marrow (erythropoietic) or liver (hepatic). The porphyrin intermediates that accumulate are responsible for the photosensitivity.

Cardinal symptoms of an ectopic pregnancy[11]

- A missed period (possibly confused with spotting at period time)
- Symptoms of pregnancy (breast tenderness, morning sickness)
- Abdominal pain, initially lower before becoming generalized
- Referred pain to shoulder tip
- Faintness and dizziness

Causes of unexpected abdominal pain following a laparotomy[11]

- Small bowel obstruction
- Pancreatitis
- Leakage from bowel anastomosis
- Perforation of viscus
- Intraperitoneal haemorrhage
- Mesenteric thrombosis
- Bile leak from biliary peritonitis
- Cholecystitis from gallstones or acalculus cholecystitis or anaemia

APPENDICITIS

Common acute surgical condition

- Incidence: M = F
- Age rare <5 years, peak incidence 10–20 years, decreasing with age thereafter
- Cause unknown
- Mucus or foreign body plug obstructing lumen
- Resulting inflammatory process purulent, gangrenous, perforation with peritonitis

Clinical features

- Malaise
- Nausea, anorexia, c/o central abdominal pain, localizing to right iliac fossa increase pain on movement or coughing
- Flushed, fetor, febrile
- Tachycardic
- Right iliac fossa localized peritonitis (may become generalized)

Investigations

Note: clinical diagnosis (investigations cannot exclude appendicitis)

- FBC, U&E
- MSU/pregnancy test

Differential diagnosis

- Mesenteric adenitis
- Gastroenteritis (common in children)
- Meckel's diverticulum, (inflammation of) Resect if inflamed or >2 cm in length or <2 cm width
- Terminal ileitis
- ?Crohn's
- UTI, cystitis
- Salpingitis
- Ruptured ectopic pregnancy
- Ruptured ovarian cyst
- Torsion of ovarian cyst

Management

- If Diagnosis is not obvious
  - Admit, observe NBM, ivi. Surgery if failure to resolve or deterioration in abdominal pain
    - Appendicectomy via Lanz, gridiron, midline incision as appropriate

Complications

General – wound infection/chest infection, DVT/PE

Specific

- Immediate
  - Bleeding from meso – appendix
  - Perforation/damage to caecum
- Short-term – pelvic abscess
- Long-term
  - Adhesions
  - Occlusion of Fallopian tubes leading to infertility

CHOLECYSTITIS/GALLSTONES

- Common (10% of population), F>M
- Cholecystitis df – inflammatory process within gallbladder wall
- May manifest with acute or chronic inflammation or complications thereof

Risk factors

- Diet
- Hypercholestrolaemia
- Multipaous women
- Drugs, e.g. OCP, clofibrate
- Haemolytic disease, e.g. Sickle cell
- TPN
- Post-truncal vagotomy
- Post-terminal ileum resection

Pathology

- Stones composition
  - Cholesterol
  - Calcium bilirubinate
  - Calcium phosphate
- 90% mixed, 5% cholesterol, 5% pigment (more common in the Far East)
- Morphology variable – solitary large, multifaceted small, sludge
- Formation
  - Metabolic (increased serum cholesterol, decreased bile salts promotes precipitation)
  - Infection
  - Biliary stasis

Complications

Gallbladder

- Acute cholecystitis
  - Perforation resulting in peritonitis
  - Gangrene
  - Empyema of gallbladder
  - Mucocele of gallbladder
  - Fistula to bowel, may cause impacted obstruction
- Chronic cholecystitis – Ca gallbladder (rare)

Biliary system

- Biliary colic
- Obstructive jaundice
  - Stone in common bile duct
  - Mirrizzi syndrome (stone in neck of gallbladder compressing common bile duct)
- Ascending cholangitis (rare)
- Pancreatitis

Indications for surgery

None – asymptomatic (incidental finding) gallstones (80%), no indication for surgery

Relative

- Persistent right upper quadrant pain (chronic cholecystitis)
- Recurrent attacks of acute cholecystitis
- Complications of gallstones, as above
- Dyspepsia to fatty foods (though exclude other causes first)

Emergency

- Generalized peritonitis
- Non-resolving acute cholecystitis or complications of

Preoperative assessment

General

- FBC, U&E, (glucose, sickle screen)
- CXR, ECG

Specific

- LFTs – note raised Br or alkaline phosphatase
- USS liver/GB/biliary tree
  - Confirm presence of gallstones
  - Note size of CBD (<7 mm)
  - Presence of dilatation of other ducts
  - Thickening or inflammatory changes of gallbladder wall

Surgical approaches

- Laparoscopic versus open cholecystectomy

'Benefits' of laparoscopic surgery

- Multiple small incisions against large subcostal incision
  - Less postoperative pain
  - Faster postoperative mobilization
    - Reduced risk of chest infection, DVT
    - Reduced hospital stay
- Cosmetic

'Risks' of laparoscopic surgery

Induction of pneumoperitoneum

- Visceral damage
  - Bowel
  - Vascular air embolism
- Bleeding from abdominal wall vessels

Diathermy

- Capacitance damage to viscera
- Damage to biliary structures via heat conductance

- No proven evidence from controlled clinical trials confirming advantage of laparoscopic method (Sheffield study).
- Incidence of major complications reported from laparoscopic surgery decreasing with experience.

- Conversion from laparoscopic to open rate falling with improved experience and better patient selection.

Relative contra-indications to laparoscopic surgery

Caution should be expressed in the following instances:
- Previous abdominal surgery
  - Risk of adhesions
  - Difficult anatomy
- Acute cholecystitis or pancreatitis
  - Obscuration of tissue planes and anatomy definition
  - Risk of sepsis through inadequate wound toilet
  - Increased bleeding from inflamed tissues
- Pre-existing cardiac or respiratory problems – may not tolerate pneumoperitoneum for long periods

When to convert laparoscopic to open
- Always convert early if problems encountered
- Uncontrollable bleeding
- Impossible to clearly define Calot's triangle (cystic duct, common hepatic duct, liver edge) or aberrant anatomy
- Rupture of gallbladder (if inflamed)
- Damage to other structures

Complications of biliary surgery

General
- Early – chest infection, Wound infection, DVT/PE
- Late – incisional hernia

Specific
- Early
  - Incorrectly applied or loosened ties/clips
  - Bleeding from cystic artery
  - Leakage from cystic duct
  - Damage to common bile duct or right hepatic duct
- Late – strictures of biliary system

May require reconstructive surgery with 'Roux-en-Y' ileal anastomosis to hepatic hilum.

COMMON BILE DUCT STONES

- Definitive diagnosis via cholangiogram
  - Endoscopic retrograde cholangiopancreatogram (ERCP)
  - Intraoperative cholangiogram (IOC)

    also

  - Percutaneous transhepatic cholangiogram (PTC)
  - Magnetic resonance cholangiopancreatogram (MRCP)

If Patients need a ERCP or IOC

- History of jaundice, dark urine, pale stools
- Gallstone pancreatitis
- Abnormal LFTs (raised Br or alkaline phosphatase)
- Dilated CBD (>7 mm) or biliary system on USS

Options

- Preoperative ERCP with spincterotomy or exploration; then open or laparoscopic chole-cystectomy
- Open cholecystectomy and IOC; exploration of CBD if required
- Laparoscopic cholecystectomy and IOC; exploration of CBD if required

TIMING OF SURGERY

Chronic cholecystitis

- Elective

Acute cholecystitis

- Non-resolving
  - >7 days without evidence of resolution
  - Empyema
  - Stone impaction in Hartmann's pouch or due to mucocele obstruction
  - Requires surgery urgently on this admission
- Resolved
  - This admission or electively
  - Elective (delayed) surgery is technically easier due to decreased inflammatory tissue
  - Urgent (early) surgery reduces risk of recurrent attacks, or complications of gallstones

Gallstone pancreatitis

as above

Peritonitis/bowel obstruction

- Rupture or gangrene of gallbladder
- Small bowel obstruction (gallstone ileus)
- Emergency surgery

PANCREATITIS

Acute – rapid onset severe inflammatory condition of pancreas associated with raised serum pancreatic enzymes, leading to local complications and potentially systemic disorder.

Chronic – continuous inflammatory disease of the pancreas, associated with irreversible structural and functional damage.

Incidence 5/100,000 UK, M = F, peak at 30–40 years of age.

Aetiology

Frequency and causes of acute pancreatitis [9]

Frequent (80–90%)

- Alcoholism

- Cholelithiasis
- Idiopathic (10%)

Occasional (10–15%)

- Postoperative pancreatitis
- Trauma
- Penetrating peptic ulcer
- Drugs (thiazides, sulphonamides, azathioprine)
- Virus (mumps, infectious mononucleosis)
- Hypercalcaemia
- Hyperlipidaemia
- Ampullary obstruction

Rare (<10%)

- Connective tissue disease
- Oestrogens
- Hypothermia
- Malnutrition – afferent loop syndrome
- Translumbar aortography

Pathology

- Initiation of autodigestion of pancreatic tissues by enzymes postinsult. Self-limiting or fulminant leading to complications and death.

Clinical presentation of acute pancreatitis

Signs and symptoms	Percentage of cases %
Abdominal pain	90
Nausea or vomiting	70
Fever	70
Abdominal distension/ascites	60
Shock	20
Dyspnoea	20
Confusion/coma	10
Cullen's or Gray–Turner's sign	<5
Subcutaneous fat necrosis	<2

Complications of acute pancreatitis

Local

- Pancreatic
  - Phlegmon
  - Pseudocyst
  - Abscess
  - Ascites
  - Haemorrhage
- Intestinal
  - Paralytic ileus
  - Gastrointestinal haemorrhage

Hepatobiliary
- Jaundice
- Obstruction of the common bile duct
- Portal vein thrombosis
- Fat necrosis

Systemic
- Metabolic
  - < Malnutrition
  - Hypocalcaemia
  - Hyperglycaemia
- Haematological
  - Disseminated intravascular coagulation
  - Portal vein thrombosis
- Renal – acute renal failure
- Cardiovascular – circulatory failure (shock)
- Respiratory – hypoxic acute respiratory failure

Investigations

Biochemistry
- Amylase, U&E, glucose, LFTs, bone
  - Amylase raised well above normal limits is diagnostic with above clinical features
  - Renal, liver function, calcium
  - Deranged glycaemic control

Haematology
- FBC, PT/PTT
  - Raised haematocrit (dehydration), leucocytosis
  - Clotting derangement
- Arterial blood gas
  - Oxygen tension
  - Systemic alkalosis (early) acidosis (late)

Radiology
- CXR – exclude perforation
- AXR
  - calcified pancreas, air within pancreatic tissue
  - fluid opacities
- USS/CT (non-urgent)
  - confirms diagnosis
  - indication to extent of damage and local complications
- ECG – may show inverted T-waves in chest leads

Management
- Resuscitate the patient
- Prevent the development of systemic disorders
- Limit the inflammatory process to reduce local complications
- High flow oxygen
- Fluid replacement
  - Colloid to maintain intravascular volume

- Crystalloid to replace sequestered fluid, extra- and intracellular volume
- Minimum 4–6 litres/24 h
- Monitoring
  - Temperature, pulse, BP, RR, O_2 saturation, urine output, blood sugar
  - CVP line, catheter, cardiac and s-monitoring
  - Saturation monitor
- Antibiotics – controversial – prevention of systemic sepsis versus preselection of organisms
- H_2 antagonists – of no proven benefit

Outcome

- Complete resolution on conservative management. No local or systemic sequelae
- Local complications
  - Conservative or minimally invasive intervention
  - Surgical intervention
- Systemic complications – resolution following systemic support
- Deterioration resulting in death

Prognosis

Numerous prognostic indicator tables devised e.g.
Ranson's criteria

- On presentation
  - Age >55 years
  - WCC >16,000/cm³
  - Glucose >11.2 mmol/l
  - LDH >350 m/l
  - SGOT >25 m

- Within 48 h
  - Haematocrit >10% rise
  - BUN >1.8 ml/l rise
  - Ca <2.0 mmol/l
  - pO_2 <7.95 kPa
  - Base deficit >4 mmol
  - Fluid loss >estimated at 6 litres

Criteria Number of Ranson's	% mortality
<3/11	<1
3–4/11	18
5–6/11	50
>6	90

Non-pancreatic causes of hyperamylasaemia[9]

- Acute and chronic renal failure
- Salivary gland disease
- Liver disease
- Gastrointestinal disease
  - Common duct stones
  - Acute cholecystitis

- Penetrating peptic ulcer
- Intestinal obstruction
- Crohn's disease
- Mesenteric infarction
- Diabetic ketoacidosis
- Gynaecological disorders
- Intracranial pathology
- Macroamylasaemia

UPPER GASTROINTESTINAL HAEMORRHAGE

Causes of upper gastrointestinal haemorrhage[13]

(Approximate frequency in brackets)

- Gastric and duodenal ulcers (50%)
- Acute gastric ulcer and erosions (20%)
- Varices (5–10%)
- Mallory–Weiss syndrome (5–10%)
- Reflux oesophagitis (5%)
- Drugs, alcohol
- Uncommon causes:
  - Gastric carcinoma
  - Hereditary telangiectasia (Osler–Weber–Rendu syndrome)
  - Pseudo xanthoma elasticum
  - Blood dyscrasias
  - Dieulafoy gastric vascular abnormality

Management

- Resuscitation and assessment
  - Oxygen
  - Intravenous access plus central line
    - Fluid crystalloid plus colloid
    - Blood
    - FFP
    - Transfusion as necessary
  - Monitoring – pulse, BP, RR, urine output, CVP
  - Check
    - FBC, U&E, clotting
    - Cross-match 6 units

If the patient is stable post–1st bleed

- Monitor and resuscitate as appropriate
- Urgent (<12 h) upper gastrointestinal endoscopy

Patient unstable despite resuscitation (i.e. evidence that bleed is continuing)

- Emergency upper gastrointestinal endoscopy
  - Diagnostic – aetiology and severity of disease
  - Therapeutic – injection of ulcer or varices

Endoscopic	Clinical
Visible vessel (50% rebleed)	Shock (systolic <90 mmHg)
Clot in ulcer base	Haemoglobin <8 g/dl
Black/red spots	Haematemesis
Left gastric artery location	Age >60 years
Gastroduodenal artery location	

Treatment
Endoscopic injection or surgical under running of a bleeding vessel

Criteria for possible surgical intervention

- Surgically treatable cause identified via endoscopy first
- Patient remains unstable despite 8 units blood (6 units if the patient is <65 years of age)
- Second major rebleed in <48 h

Surgical treatment for a Bleeding ulcer

- Partial Gastrectomy or/gastrostomy plus undersewing of ulcer

Factors predisposing to rebleeding

Causes of acute gastric erosions

- Burns (Curling's ulcers)
- Head injury (Cushing's ulcer)
- Major trauma
- Sepsis
- MOF
- Alcohol, NSAIDs, etc.

Treatment

- Pharmacological acid suppression or sulcaphate

Oesophageal varices

- 90% occurs within 2 cm of the gastro-oesophageal junction
- Long-term survival is related to Child's classification of liver disease (see page ???)

Treatment

- Sengstaken–Blakemore tube
  - Gastric balloon filled with 200 ml water and tamponades the bleeding temporarily
  - Oesophageal balloon, if required, is inflated to no more than the mean arterial pressure and is released every 2 h to prevent ulceration
- Intravariceal sclerotherapy – with ethanolamine oleate
- Vasopressin/somatostatin – both lower portal pressure
- Portosystemic shunts
  - The more proximal the shunt, the more effective it is, but the greater the risk of hepatic encephalopathy
  - Shunts should be considered after two failed sessions of sclerotherapy
- Transjugular intrahepatic portosystemic anastomosis (TIPS) are performed radiologically
- Oesophageal transection, devascularization and stapled reanastomosis via a gastrostomy has a high operative mortality rate

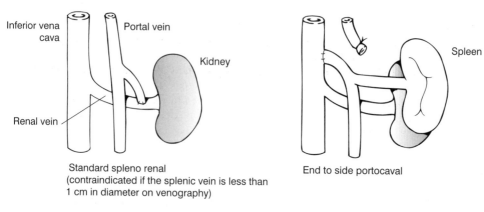

Standard spleno renal
(contraindicated if the splenic vein is less than
1 cm in diameter on venography)

End to side portocaval

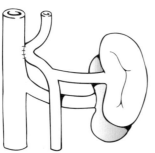

Side to side porto canal
(lowest incidence of encephalopathy)

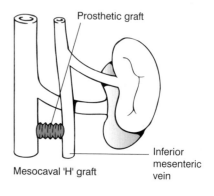

Mesocaval 'H' graft

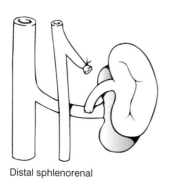

Distal sphlenorenal

Figure 5.1 Main types of portosystemic shunts.

Other causes of gastrointestinal haemorrhage

- Mallory–Weiss tear – 90% usually resolve spontaneously. Occurs at lesser curve gastro-oesophageal junction in 80% of cases.
- Aortic enteric fistula should be considered in all patients with an aortic graft. There is usually a small 'herald' bleed preceding the major haematemesis.
- Gastric leiomyoma – the commonest tumour to produce a major gastrointestinal bleed. It appears as a yellowish polyp with an ulcerated crater and is cured by local excision. Gastric carcinoma ooze slowly.

OESOPHAGUS

FACTORS IN MAINTAINING COMPETENCE OF THE OESOPHAGEAL-GASTRIC JUNCTION

- Intrinsic functional lower oesophageal sphincter.
- Length of intra-abdominal oesophagus compressed by the positive (intra-abdominal) pressure of the abdomen, its lumen being at negative intrathoracic pressure.
- Pinch-cock effect of right crus of the diaphragm on the intra-abdominal oesophagus
- Oblique insertion of the oesophagus into the stomach creating the Angle of His.

OESOPAGHEAL DISORDERS

Trauma
- Spontaneous Boorhaave's syndrome
  - Treatment
    - Early surgical repair or
    - Conservative
      - Chest drain plus feeding jejunostomy
      - Healing 6 weeks
- Mortality rate of 10%
- Penetrating
- Iatrogenic (instrumentation)

Oesophagitis
Gastro-oesophageal reflux
- Causes/risk factors
  - Smoking/alcohol/obesity
  - Hiatus hernia
    - Sliding
    - Paraoesophageal
- Complications
  - Barret's metaplasia
  - Incarceration/volvulus hiatus hernia
  - Ulceration

- Treatment
  - Conservative (reduce smoking, drinking, weight)
  - Antacids, H_2 antagonists, proton pump blockers
  - Fundoplication

Achalasia

- Incidence 1/100,000, 30–60 years of age
- Aetiology Motility disorder of distal oesophagus? Deficiency in Auerbach's plexus
- Dysphagia and regurgitation, liquids > solids
- Investigation 'Birds beak oesophagus' on radiology
- Treatment:
  - Oesophageal balloon dilatation (70% success rate, 3% perforation rate)
  - Surgical cardiomyotomy
- Consider Chagas' disease, Tryponosoma cruzi aganglionosis

Scleroderma

- Aetiology
  - CREST syndrome
  - Adynamic oesophagus

Diffuse oesophageal spasm

- Nutcracker oesophagus
- Diagnoses on oesophageal manometry

Treatment

- Balloon dilation or myotomy

Diverticula

- Aetiology Congenital
- Pulsion
- Traction (e.g. TB)

Premalignant lesions of the oesophagus

- Plummer–Vinson syndrome (chronic iron deficiency in women with oesophageal webs predisposing to postcricoid carcinoma)
- Achalasia of the cardia
- Corrosive oesophagitis
- Gastro-oesophageal reflux (leading to peptic stricture and Barrett's oesophagitis)

Oesophageal carcinoma

- incidence 4000 deaths p.a. in the UK
- 5% of malignancies
- Age >45 years, with an increasing incidence with age
- M>F

Risk factors

- Smoking
- Alcohol
- Nitrosamines, including those present in the diet
- Decreased vitamins C and A in the diet
- Familial
- Premalignant lesions
  - Webs
  - Peptic strictures
  - Achalasia
  - Barrett's metaplasia

Clinical features

- Dysphagia
  - Progressive
  - Solids > liquids
- Weight loss
- Regurgitation and aspiration
- Pain

Pathology

- Upper 2/3 squamous cell carcinoma (90%)
- Lower 1/3 adenocarcinoma (10%)
- Lesions
  - Annular stenosing
  - Ulcer-like
  - Fungating cauliflower-like

Spread

Direct
- Submucosal and transmucosal
- Invasion of mediastinal structures
- Trachea and bronchus – fistula and pneumonia
- Recurrent laryngeal nerve – hoarse voice
- Aorta – bleed
- Direct perforation – mediastinitis

Lymph
- Local – submucosal spread
- Distant
  - Cervical – supraclavicular fossa
  - Thoracic
    - Paraoesophageal nodes
    - Tracheobronchial nodes
  - Abdominal
    - Lesser curve of stomach nodes
    - Coeliac axis

Blood – liver

Investigations
- Upper gastrointestinal endoscopy plus biopsy
- CT scan thorax plus abdomen to assess extent

Stage
- **I** – mucosa/submucosa +, serosa/node –
- **II** – serosa + node –
- **III** – node +
- **IV** – distant metastases

Management

Curative (25% of cases are suitable)
- Disease localized to oesophagus only
- No local lymph node or disseminated disease
- Patient fit to undergo major treatment
  - Squamous cell carcinoma – high-dose curative radiotherapy
  - Adenocarcinoma
    - Oesophageal resection
    - Lower/middle oesophagus
    - Ivor Lewis procedure
      - Two-stage oesphagogastrectomy
      - Lower oesophagus
        - Mobilized via midline abdominal incision
        - Oesophagus resected via right thoracotomy
    - Upper oesophagus
      - McKeown three stage oesophagectomy
      - As above, plus complete mobilization of thoracic oesophagus
      - Anastomosis with cervical oesophagus via neck incision

Complications of surgery
- Mortality rate of 15%
- Anastomotic leak
- Chest infection
- Mediastinitis
- Reflux symptoms
- General complications of major surgery
- Oesophagectomy covered with feeding jejunostomy until a satisfactory recovery is achieved

Prognosis
- Overall 45% 1YS
- 15% 5YS
- Palliative treatment is indicated in 75% of cases
- Limit symptoms of dysphagia and weight loss
- 50% mortality rate at 6 months
  - Endoscopic intubation plus prosthetic stent
  - Laser photocoagulation
  - Electrodiathermy
  - Photodynamic therapy

Complications of endoscopic procedures

- Oesophageal perforation
- Stent migration
- Tumour overgrowth
- Reflux

No evidence of benefit from adjuvant chemotherapy.

STOMACH AND DUODENUM

PEPTIC ULCER DISEASE

- Mucosal ulceration presence of acid secretion
- Common M>F
- Duodenum
- Stomach

also

- Lower oesophagus
- Gastric mucosa within Meckel's
- Stoma post gastrojejunostomy

Risk factors

- Infection with *Helicobacter pylori*
- Smoking
- Alcohol
- Drugs NSAIDs, aspirin, steroids
- Gastrin-secreting tumours (Zollinger–Ellison syndrome)
- Genetic
- Stress

Complications

Acute

- Perforation
- Haematesis

Chronic

- Pyloric stenosis
- Hourglass contrature
- Penetration into neighbouring viscera
- Carcinoma (gastric)

Clinical features

- Epigastric pain
- Nausea
  - Gastric
    - On eating
    - Relived by milk/antacids

- Weight loss
- Risk of malignant transformation
- Duodenal
- 2–3 h postprandial
- Nocturnal pain

Management
- Primarily medical
  - Reduce or eliminate risk factors (e.g. change medication)
  - Eradicate *H. pylori*
  - Suppress acid secretion
    - Triple therapy (proton pump blocker plus antibiotic × 2) – 1 week
    - Dual therapy (H_2 antagonist and antibiotic) – 2 weeks
    - Continue anti-acid medication – 6–8 weeks
- Surgery
  - Complications acute/chronic
  - Failure of medical management
  - Possibility of malignancy
  - Bilroth II gastrectomy
  - Vagotomy and antrectomy (see page 97) (rare)

GASTRIC CANCER

- Incidence >10,000 deaths/year, 60/100,000 in the UK (a rate that is decreasing)
- Peak incidence 60–75-year age group, M>F = 1.5:1
- Highest incidence in Japan, China and South America

Risk factors
- Dietary nitrate (smoked foods)/food preservatives
- Smoking
- Alcohol
- Mining/pottery industry (the UK incidence is high in South Wales and the Midlands)
- Genetic (?blood group A)

Premalignant lesions/associations
- Gastric polyps
- Atrophic gastritis
- Pernicious anaemia
- Postgastrectomy/vagotomy
- Biliary reflux gastritis
- Hypochlorhydria (acid suppression)
- *H. pylori*

Clinical features
- Insidious onset
- Dyspepsia, bloating, epigastric pain
- Weight loss, anorexia, malaise
- Dysphagia/signs of metastatic disease (late)

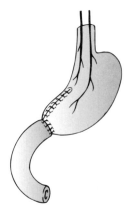

Figure 5.2b Surgical treatment for benign gastric ulcers.

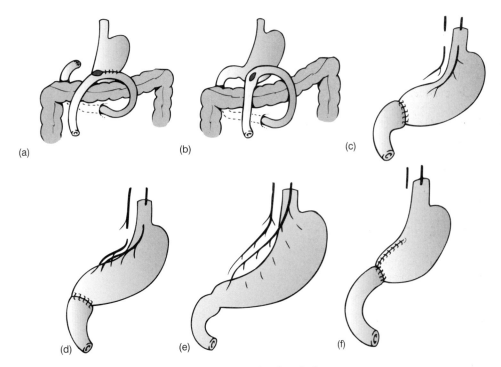

Figure 5.2a Surgical treatment for benign duodenal ulcers.

Investigations

- Upper gastrointestinal endoscopy plus biopsy
- CT scan thorax/abdomen to assess stage
- Laparoscopy
- Endoluminal USS

Pathology

Lesions – ulcerating, polyploidal or diffuse (leather bottle)

- Pylorus/prepyloric region (50%)
- Lesser curve (25%)
- Cardia (10%)
- Multifocal (15%)
- Adenocarcinoma (90%)
- Other (SCC, Lymphoma) (10%)
- Leiomyosarcoma, carcinoid

Spread

- Direct – invasion to pancreas, transverse colon, oesophagus, liver
- Lymph nodes
  - N1 perigastric nodes <3 cm from lesion
  - N2 >3 cm lesion, along L/R gastric, gastroepiploic, splenic nodes
  - N3 distant – porta hepatis, infracolic, preaortic
- Blood – liver, lung, bone, skin
- Transcoelomic – peritoneum, ovary (Krukenberg tumours)

Stage

TNM clinical classification of stomach cancer

T – primary tumour

- **Tx** – primary tumour cannot be assessed
- **T0** – no evidence of primary tumour
- **Tis** – carcinoma *in situ* – intraepithelial tumour without invasion of lamina propria
- **T1** – tumour invades lamina propria and submucosa
- **T2** – tumour invades muscularis propria and submucosa A
- **T3** – tumour penetrates serosa (visceral peritoneum) without invasion of adjacent structures A, B and C
- **T4** – tumour invades adjacent structures B and C

N – regional lymph nodes

- **Nx** – regional lymph nodes cannot be assessed
- **N0** – no regional lymph nodes metastasis
- **N1** – metastasis in perigastric lymph node(s) (1-6)
- **N2** – metastasis in perigastric lymph node(s) (7-15)
- **N3** – Metatasis in more than 15 regional lymph nodes
- **A** – a tumour may penetrate the muscularis propria with extension into the gastrocolic or gastrohepatic ligaments, or the greater or lesser omentum without perforation of the visceral peritoneum covering these structures. In this case, the tumour is classified as T2. If there is perforation of the visceral peritoneum covering the gastric ligaments or omentum. the tumour is classified as T3

- **B** –adjacent structures of the stomach are the spleen, transverse colon, liver, diaphragm, pancreas, abdominal wall, adrenal gland, kidney, small intestine and retroperitoneum
- **C** – intramural extension to the duodenum or oesophagus is classified by the depth of greater invasion in any of these sites including the stomach

The more commonly used is stage:

- **I** – mucosa/submucosa +, serosa/node –
- **II** – serosa +, node –
- **III** – node +
- **IV** – distant metastasis or nodes (N3)

Treatment

- More radical surgery practised in Japan (stages I–III)
- The UK is more likely to treat stages I–II only curatively
- Later presentation in the UK has a lesser rate of curative surgery practised

Curative surgery

Gastrectomy

- Tumour plus omentum with at least 3 cm resection margins
  - Pyloric tumours – partial gastrectomy (Bilroth II)
  - Body/fundus tumours – total gastrectomy

Lymph node dissection

- D1 resection of N1 nodes
- D2 N1 + N2 nodes dissected

Palliative treatment

- Symptomatic relief – gastrojejunostomy or feeding tube

Prognosis

- Japan – D2 gastrectomy is normally practised producing claims of is for >80% 5YS versus 40% for D1 gastrectomy
- UK – high morbidity associated with D2 gastrectomy
- No overall difference in survival figures, D1 gastrectomy mostly carried out
- Overall 20% 5YS
- Late presentation UK versus Japan (screening programme, dedicated units)

Stage	5 Year Survival (5YS)
I	75%
II	45%
III	25%
IV	<5%

Adjuvant treatment

- No proven benefit of postoperative adjuvant chemotherapy in curative resection
- MAGIC trial at present to assess preoperative chemotherapy
- Reported response rate to cisplatinum in advanced disease (but not improving survival figures)

Specific complications postgastrectomy

Early

- Bleeding from anastomosis (very vascular)
- Anastomotic leak
- Duodenal stump blow-out
- Stomal obstruction
  - Oedema
  - Retrograde jejunogastric intussusseption
  - Atonic stomach
- Postoperative pancreatitis
- Early postgastrectomy syndromes (dumping)
  - Post-ingestion abdominal pain, nausea, sweating, tachycardia (vasomotor)
  - Owing to rapid passage of carbohydrate into small bowel
  - Transient hyperglycaemia then hypoglycaemia (increased insulin sensitivity)
  - Improves with time
  - Advise small, frequent meals

Late

- Late postgastrectomy syndromes (nutritional disorders)
  - Weight loss
  - Steathorrea
  - Diarrhoea
  - Iron deficiency anaemia
  - Megaloblastic anaemia
  - Vitamin B deficiency
  - Calcium deficiency
  - Malabsorption
- Recurrent carcinoma

SPLEEN, LIVER AND PANCREAS

ORGANS SOMETIME PALPABLE IN THIN SUBJECTS

- Liver (10%)
- Spleen should not be felt
- Aorta
- Left kidney (7%)
- Lower pole right kidney (15%)
- Sigmoid colon (75%)

CAUSES OF HEPATOMEGALY[12]

- Smooth, generalized enlargement, without jaundice
  - Congestion from heart failure

- Cirrhosis
- Reticuloses
- Hepatic vein obstruction (Budd–Chiari syndrome)
- Amyloid disease
- Knobbly generalized enlargement, without jaundice
  - Secondary carcinoma
  - Macronodular cirrhosis
  - Polycyclic disease
  - Primary liver carcinoma
- Knobbly generalizes enlargement, with jaundice
  - Extensive secondary carcinoma
  - Cirrhosis
- Smooth generalized enlargement, with jaundice
  - Infective hepatitis
  - Biliary tract obstruction (gallstones, carcinoma of the pancreas)
  - Cholangitis
  - Portal pyaemia
- Localized swellings
  - Riedel's lobe
  - Secondary carcinoma
  - Hydatid cyst
  - Liver abscess
- Primary liver carcinoma

CAUSES OF SPLENOMEGALY (AND THE MORE COMMON INDICATIONS FOR SPLENECTOMY* EXCLUDING TRAUMA)[12]

Infection

Bacterial
- Typhoid
- Typhus
- Tuberculosis
- General septicaemia

Spirochaetal
- Syphilis
- Leptospirosis (Weil's disease)

Viral – glandular fever

Protozoal
- Malaria
- Kala-azar

Cellular proliferation

- Myeloid and lymphatic leukaemia
- Pernicious anaemia
- Haemolytic (autoimmune) anaemia*
- Polycythaemia anaemia
- Spherocytosis (hereditary)
- Thrombocytopenic purpura (ITP)*

- Myelosclerosis
- Mediterranean anaemia

Congestion

- Portal hypertension★ (cirrhosis, portal vein thrombosis)
- Hepatic vein obstruction
- Congestive heart failure (cor pulmonale, constrictive pericarditis)

Infarction

- Embolic★ from bacterial endocarditis, emboli from the left atrium during atrial fibrillation associated with mitral stenosis, emboli from the left ventricle after myocardial infarction
- Splenic artery or vein thrombosis in polycythaemia and retroperitoneal malignancy

Cellular infiltration

- Amyloidosis
- Gaucher's disease★

Collagen diseases

- Felty's syndrome
- Still's disease

Space-occupying lesions

- True solitary cysts
- Polycystic disease
- Hydatid cysts
- Angioma
- Lymphosarcoma

Lymphoma

N.B. Splenectomy is sometimes indicated during other surgical procedures (e.g. gastric cancer, distal pancreatechomy and portal decompression).

COMPLICATIONS OF SPLENECTOMY

- Haemorrhage
- Pulmonary atelectasis
- Subphrenic abscess
- Post-splenectomy fever
- Thrombocytosis (increased platelets leading to DVT and PE)
- Overwhelming sepsis (prophylaxis polyvalent pneumococcal vaccine and penicillin V)
- Pancreatic fistula
- Gastric fistula
- Splenunculi

LIVER MALIGNANCY

- Primary
  - Hepatocellular carcinoma
  - Cholangiocarcinoma

- Secondary
  - Gastrointestinal tract
  - Urogenital tract
  - Breast/prostate
  - Carcinoid

HEPATOCELLULAR CARCINOMA

- Rare in the UK, though common in the Far East
- Background cirrhotic liver
- Lesions single or multicentric
- Variation in speed of progression – spread to lymph nodes, mediastinum, neck
- Symptoms
  - Anorexia, weight loss
  - Hepatomegaly/mass
- Investigations
  - α-Fetoprotein (AFP) elevated early in disease
  - USS/CT plus biopsy
- Treatment – (untreated – mean survival = 3–6 months)
- Localized lesion
- Consider hemihepatectomy
- Hepatic artery chemotherapy
- Liver transplantation

CHOLANGIOCARCINOMA

- Rare
- Risk factor
- Ulcerative colitis, primary sclerosing cholangitis, choledochal cyst, Caroli disease
- Symptoms
  - Obstructive jaundice, biliary pain, cholangitis
  - Weight loss, anorexia
- Investigations – LFTs, CT/MRCP
- Treatment – ERCP plus biopsy (plus stent)
- Depends on area of lesion
  - Hilar region (50%)
    - Non-surgical
    - Stenting – endoscopic/percutaneous
    - +/– Radio Tx
  - Lower duct system – resection w Roux-en-Y
- Overall poor prognosis
- Mainly palliative procedures only

SECONDARY LIVER TUMOURS

- Most common liver neoplasm
- Disseminated disease, most cases palliative treatment only
- Solitary liver lesion consider, resection + intra-arterial chemotherapy

CLASSIFICATION OF PRIMARY MALIGNANT TUMOURS OF THE PANCREAS (99.5% MALIGNANT)[9]

Origin	Type of tumour
Ductal epithelium	Carcinoma – adenocarcinoma, giant cell, adenosquamous, mucinous, microadenocarcinoma, cystadenocarcinoma, papillary cystic tumour, unclassified
Acinar cells	Acinar cell carcinoma
Islet cells	Malignant insulinoma, gastrinoma, VIPoma, glucagonoma, and others
Non- epithelial tissue	Fibrosarcoma, leiomyosarcoma, haemangiopericytoma, histiocytoma, lymphoma[11]

Epidemiology

- 12/100,000 p.a., [ss]6000 deaths p.a.
- Increasing incidence or earlier diagnosis
- M = F approximately
- 50% patients are >70 years of age at diagnosis

Pathology

- Head and neck > body and tail 2:1
- Adenocarcinoma – 19% with local duct cell carcinoma *in situ*
- Cyst adenocarcinoma – large cystic lesions, less aggressive

Spread

- Local invasion
- SMV, HPV, liver
- Para-aortic/mesenteric lymph nodes

Risk factors

- Smoking
- Diet (high fat and protein)
- Alcohol secondary to chronic pancreatitis

Clinical features[14]

Symptom	Ampulla (%)	Head/neck (%)	Body/tail (%)
Weight loss	62	83	71
Pain	38	48	90
Jaundice	77	65	0
Painless jaundice	46	27	0
Anorexia	69	44	52
Thrombophlebitis	8	8	9.5

TNM classification of pancreatic carcinomas[7]

T – primary tumour

- **T1** – no direct extension of primary tumour beyond the pancreas, <2cm in size
- **T2** – limited to pancreas, >2cm in greatest dimension
- **T3** – limited direct extension to duodenum, bile duct, or stomach
- **T4** – advanced direct extension precluding surgical resection

N – regional lymph node

- **N0** – regional nodes not involved
- **N1** – regional nodes involved

M – distant metastases

- **M0** – no distant metastasis
- **M1** – distant metastasis

Stage grouping of pancreatic carcinomas[7]

Stage	TNM classification		
I	T1, T2	N0	M0
II	T3	N0	M0
III	T1, T2, T3	N1	M0
IV	T4	N0, N1	M1

Decision tree for management of patients with pancreatic carcinoma[7]

- Suspected pancreatic cancer
- CT scan or ultrasound
- Advanced disease >80% cases. Advanced age of patients
- 95% palliative treatment
  - Jaundice
    - Stent
    - Surgical biliary bypass
  - Duodenal obstruction Gastroenterostomy
- 5% Surgical resection
  - <5 cm diameter
    - Localized to head/neck
    - No disseminated disease
  - Whipple's procedure (pancreatoduodenectomy)

Prognosis

- Overall 50% survival at 6 months
- 3% survive for 5 years

Surgical resection

- 15% operative mortality rate
- Up to 30% 5-year survival rate

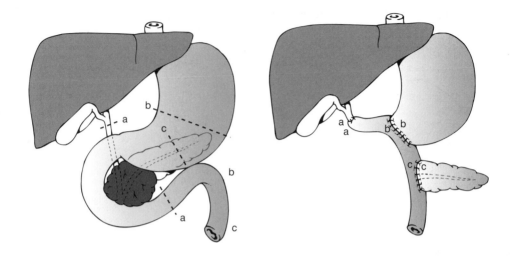

Figure 5.3 Management of extrahepatic cholangiocarcinoma, ampullary pancreatic and duodenal carcinoma – pancreaticoduodenectomy (Whipple's operation). Structures are divided at the dotted lines (removing the distal half of the stomach, entire duodenal loop, the body of the pancreas and the lower end of the common bile duct) and are reconstructed to the proximal jejunum.

NON-MALIGNANT NEOPLASIA OF THE GASTROINTESTINAL TRACT

Liver
- Hepatocytes – hepatoma
- Bile ducts – cholangiadenoma
- Vascular – haemangioma
  - All rare, Mainly asymptomatic, Incidental findings or Pressure effect, No malignant potential, possible hepatoma link to OCP

Pancreas
- Endocrine tumours (99% benign)
  - Alpha cell tumour – Zollinger–Ellison syndrome
  - Beta cell tumour – insulinoma
  - Gamma cell tumour
- Islet cell lesion
  - Hyperplasia
  - Adenoma
    - Discrete local
    - Multifocal
  - Carcinoma
- May consist of part of a MEN type I syndrome

BETA CELL TUMOUR – INSULINOMA

- Insulin-secreting lesion
  - Intermittent episodes of hypoglycaemia
    - Abdominal pain relieved by eating (cf. duodenal ulcer)
    - Sweating, dizziness, trembling
    - Speech, visual, movement disorders
    - Seizures
- Whipple's triad
  - Clinical features, as above
  - Blood glucose <2.5 mmol/l
  - Relief via glucose infusion
- Investigations
  - Fasting hypoglycaemia plus raised serum insulin
  - CT/MRI

Treatment

- Surgical resection

ZOLLINGER–ELLISON SYNDROME

Severe, recurrent peptic ulceration, atypical sites

- ZES type I – antral G-cell hyperplasia
- ZES type II – alpha cell tumour or diffuse hyperplasia
  - Gastrin-secreting lesion
  - Associated ulceration, diarrhoea, steatorrhoea
- Investigations
  - Plasma gastrin levels
  - CT/MRI scan

Treatment

- I – partial gastrectomy
- II – excision of lesion

Gastric

- Leiomyoma
- Neurofibroma
- Adenomatous polyp
- Aberrant pancreas
- Menetrier's disease (giant hypertrophy of gastric fundal mucosa)

Small bowel

(see page 114)

MISCELLANEOUS

DISEASES OF THE UMBILICUS[14]

- Inflammations
  - Infection of the stump of the umbilical cord (omphalitis)
  - Umbilical granuloma
  - Umbilical dermatitis (intertrigo)
  - Umbilical pilonidal sinus
- Fistulas
  - Faecal
    - Patent vitello-intestinal duct (congenital)
    - Neoplastic ulceration (from the transverse colon usually)
    - Tuberculous peritonitis
  - Urinary – patent arachus (congenital)
  - Biliary
  - Neoplasms
  - Benign
    - Adenoma (raspberry tumour, congenital)
    - Endometrioma
  - Malignant
    - Primary carcinoma – stomach
    - Secondary carcinoma – colorectal, ovary and uterus, breast
- Hernia
- Umbilical calculus
- Eversion (in ascites)

MECHANISMS AND CAUSES OF ASCITES[5]

- Infection – tuberculosis, peritonitis, etc.
- Inflammatory disease – Crohn's disease, starch peritonitis
- Hypoproteinaemia – nephrotic syndrome, liver disease, protein losing enteropathy
- Lymphatic obstruction – tuberculosis, filariasis, lymphoma, metastatic carcinoma, Milroy's disease, rupture/damage of abdominal lymphatics
- Increased lymph flow/pressure – congested cardiac failure, constricted pericarditis and cirrhosis
- Portal hypertension/congestion – cirrhosis, congestive cardiac failure, constrictive peritonitis, Budd–Chiari syndrome
- Neoplasms – primary and secondary tumours of the peritoneal cavity
- Chronic pancreatitis – pancreatic ascites

Note: in many instances, the ascites is multifactorial in origin.

DISEASE OF THE PERITONEUM[13]

- Infective (bacterial) peritonitis
  - Secondary to gut disease
    - Appendicitis
    - Perforation of any organ
    - Chronic peritoneal dialysis

- – Spontaneous, usually in ascites with liver disease
- – TB
- Neoplasia
- Secondary deposits, e.g. from ovary and stomach
- Primary mesothelioma
- Vasculitis – connective tissue disease

EMBOLISM AND THROMBOSIS OF THE MESENTERIC VESSELS

- Embolism of the superior mesenteric artery. Possible sources of emboli include the left auricle (especially in atrial fibrillation), a mural myocardial infarct, an atheromatous plaque of aneurysm of the aorta, a vegetation on the mitral valve, pulmonary vein thrombosis secondary to septic infarct or a fragment from a left atrial myxoma.
- Primary thrombosis of the superior mesenteric artery is the result of either arteriosclerosis or thromboangitis obliterans.
- Primary thrombosis of the superior mesenteric vein or its tributaries occurs occasionally in portal hypertension, portal pyaemia (pylephlebitis), sickle-cell disease and in women taking the contraceptive pill.

CAUSES OF ISCHAEMIC COLITIS[5]

Thrombosis (arterial or venous)
- Arteriosclerosis
- Polycythaemia vera
- Portal hypertension
- Malignant disease of the colon
- Hyperviscosity syndrome due to:
  - Platelet abnormalities
  - High molecular weight dextran infusion

Emboli from:
- Left atrium (atrial fibrillation)
- Left ventricle (myocardial infarction)
- Atheromatous plaque in aorta

Vasculitis
- Polyarteritis nodosa
- Lupus erythematous
- Giant-cell arteritis (Takayasu's arteritis)
- Buerger's disease
- Henoch–Schonlein disease

Surgical trauma to vessels
- Aortic reconstruction
- Resection of adjacent intestine

Non-occlusive ischaemia
- Shock – hypovolaemic or septic
- Congestive heart failure

'Spontaneous' ischaemic colitis

CAUSES OF INTRAPERITONEAL ADHESIONS[5]

- Ischaemic areas – sites of anastomoses, reperitonealization of raw areas

- Foreign bodies – talc, starch granules, gauze lint, cellulose, non-absorbable sutures
- Infective disease – peritonitis, tuberculosis
- Inflammatory disease – Crohn's disease
- Radiation enteritis
- Sclerosing peritonitis – usually drug-induced (certain β-blockers, e.g. practolol)

CAUSES OF NON-MALIGNANT STRICTURES

- Congenital
- Spasmodic
- Organic
  - Postoperative stricture
  - Irradiation stricture
  - Senile anal stricture
  - Lymphogranuloma inguinale
  - Inflammatory bowel disease
  - Endometriosis
  - Neoplastic

CAUSES OF RETROPERITONEAL FIBROSIS[4]

Benign

- Idiopathic (Ormond's disease)
- Drugs
  - Methysergide (Sansert), LSD, β-agonists, amphetamines, ergot alkaloids, haloperidol, reserpine
  - Phenacetin, methyldopa (Aldomet), chemotherapeutic agents
- Infections
  - Chronic urinary tract infections
  - Tuberculosis
  - Gonorrhoea
  - Syphilis
- Non-specific inflammatory conditions
  - Collagen-vascular disease/autoimmune diseases
  - Periarteritis
  - Aortic or iliac aneurysm
  - Urinoma
- Specific inflammatory condition
  - Inflammatory conditions
  - Endometriosis
  - Sarcoidosis
  - Gastrointestinal tract infections and inflammation
- Haemorrhage
  - Trauma (leaking of blood or urine)
  - Post-surgical

Retroperitoneal malignancy

- Primary tumours – neuroblastomas, ganglioneuromas, sarcomas, lymphoma, lipoma, teratoma, adrenogenital

- Metastatic tumours – carcinoid, stomach, colon, breast, prostate
- Radiation therapy

CAUSES OF DIARRHOEA[12]

Intestinal
- Enteritis
  - Non-specific
  - Staphylococcal
  - Typhoid
  - Bacillary dysentery
  - Amoebic
  - Cholera
- Worms
- Ulcerative colitis
- Crohn's disease
- Carcinoma
- Irritable colon
- Faecal impaction (spurious diarrhoea)
- Tropical sprue

Gastric
- Postgastrectomy
- Post-vagotomy
- Gastrocolic

Pancreatic
- Pancreatitis
- Carcinoma

Pelvic abscess

Drugs
- Digitalis
- Antibiotics
- Laxatives

Endocrine
- Uraemia
- Thyrotoxicosis
- Carcinoid syndrome
- Zollinger–Ellison syndrome
- Medullary carcinoma of the thyroid
- Hypoparathyroidism
- Diet

Symptoms and signs associated with chronic diarrhoea[33]	
Symptoms and signs	**Syndrome**
Arthritis	UC, Crohn's, Whipple's disease
Liver disease	UC, Crohn's, metastases from colonic carcinoma
Fever	UC, Crohn's, amoebiasis, Whipple's, TB
Uveitis	UC, Crohn's
Pyoderma granulosa	UC
Erythema nodosum	Inflammatory bowel disease, yersinosis
Severe weight loss	Malabsorption, cancer, thyrotoxicosis, inflammatory bowel disease
Lymphadenopathy	Lymphoma, HIV, Whipple's disease,
Neuropathy	Diabetic diarrhoea, amyloidosis
Dermatitis herpetiformis	Coeliac disease
Flushing	Carcinoid

CAUSES OF CONSTIPATION[13]

- Simple
- Intestinal obstruction
- Colonic disease, e.g. carcinoma
- Painful anal conditions
- Drugs, e.g. opiates, aluminium antacids, antidepressants, codeine, iron
- Hypothyroidism, hypercalcaemia
- Depression
- Immobility
- Hirschsprung's disease (very occasionally seen in adults)

CAUSES OF A MASS IN THE RIGHT ILIAC FOSSA[12]

- Appendicitis
- TB ileum
- Carcinoma of caecum
- Intussusception
- Crohn's disease (terminal ileitis)
- Iliac lymphadenopathy
- Iliac artery aneurysm
- Psoas abscess
- Chondrosarcoma of the ilium
- Tumour in an undescended testis
- Actinomycosis
- Ruptured epigastric artery/haematoma
- Gynaecological
- Pelvic kidney
- Carcinoid tumour
- (For left iliac fossa, delete the first four causes and insert diverticulitis and carcinoma of the colon.)

AGE, AND COMMON CAUSES OF ALIMENTARY TRACT OBSTRUCTION[12]

Birth
- Atresia (duodenum, ileum)
- Meconium obstruction
- Volvulus neonatorum

3–6 weeks – congenital hypertrophic pyloric stenosis
6–18 months – intussusception

Teenage
- Inflammatory masses (appendicitis)
- Intussusception of Meckel's diverticulum or polyp

Young adult
- Hernia
- Adhesions

Adult
- Hernia
- Adhesions
- Inflammatory (appendicitis, Crohn's disease)
- Carcinoma

Elderly
- Carcinoma
- Inflammation (diverticulitis)
- Sigmoid volvulus
- Hernia

CAUSES OF PSEUDO-OBSTRUCTION

Idiopathic
Retroperitoneal irritation by:
- Blood
- Urine
- Enzymes (pancreatitis)
- Tumour

Idiosyncratic drug reaction
- Tricyclics
- Phenothiazines
- Levodopa

Metabolic disorder
- Diabetes
- Hypokalaemia
- Uraemia
- Myxoedema

Severe trauma (especially to lumbar spine and pelvis)
Shock
- Severe burns
- Myocardial infarct
- Stroke

Septicaemia

SMALL BOWEL

CAUSES OF DUODENAL OBSTRUCTION[9]

- Duodenal atresia or stenosis
- Duodenal obstruction associated with malrotation
- Annular pancreas
- Duodenal web
- Preduodenal portal vein
- Duodenal duplication cyst
- Extrinsic compression by adjacent masses

CAUSES OF SMALL BOWEL OBSTRUCTION

- Adhesions (70%)
- Hernia (20%)
- Malignancy, other (10%)
- Site – pathology
- Extrinsic – adhesions, hernia, volvulus, congenital bands, inflammatory mass
- Mural – atresia, inflammatory bowel disease, tumours, intussusception, ischaemia, TB
- Luminal – meconium, bezoars, gallstones, congenital bands, malignancy, inflammatory mass

SMALL BOWEL TUMOURS

Malignant small bowel tumours	Incidence
Adenocarcinoma (39%)	50% are duodenal (Treatment- pancreaticoduodenectomy)
Carcinoid (29%)	73% of malignant carcinoids occur in the ileum
	• Appendiceal tumours <1 cm can be cured with an appendicectomy
	• Larger lesions require a right hemicolectomy
Lymphoma (14%)	Treatment- chemotherapy, obstructing or perforating lesions can be resected
Sarcoma (14%)	
Note: <2% of gastrointestinal malignancies are small bowel and 50% are duodenal.	

NON-MALIGNANT TUMOURS OF THE SMALL INTESTINE[9]

Benign neoplasms

- Epithelial
  - Tubular adenoma
  - Villous adenoma★
  - Polyposis syndromes (adenoma)
- Brunner's gland adenoma
- Stromal
  - Adipose tissue – lipoma

- Connective tissue
  - Smooth muscle tumours
  - Neurogenic tumours
  - Fibroma
- Endothelium
  - Vascular tumours
  - Lymphatic tumours

Intermediate neoplasms (endocrine tumours)

Hamartomatous lesions

- Peutz–Jeghers syndrome
- Other polyposis syndrome (hamartoma)

Heterotopic tissue

- Localized
- Disseminated

Duplications

⋆ Villous adenoma and leiomyoma have a strong malignant potential and could also be regarded as intermediate neoplasms.

CLASSIFICATION OF MESENTERIC CYSTS

- Chylolymphatic
- Enterogenous
- Urogenital remnant
- Dermoid (teratomatous cyst)

FACTORS FAVOURING EXCISION OF AN INCIDENTAL MECKEL'S DIVERTICULUM

- Age <40 years of age
- Presence of ectopic mucosa
- Scarring or induration
- Size of base less than twice the length
- Undiagnosed rectal bleeding

CONSEQUENCES OF COMPLETE RESECTION OF ILEUM OR JEJUNUM[29]

- Function of jejunum – generalized transport of water, electrolytes, sugars, proteins, fats and vitamins. Most absorption occurs proximally.
- Function of ileum – localized transport of bile salts, cholesterol, vitamin B_{12} absorption in ileum only.
- Changes after resection of jejunum – general transport and workload assumed by ileum. Localized transport unaffected therefore no malabsorption.
- Changes after resection of ileum – generalized transport continues. Localized transport lost. Malabsorption of vitamin B_{12}, cholesterol, bile salts and fats.

> **Sequelae of massive resection or extensive by-pass of the small intestine[5]**
> - Malabsorption and malnutrition
> - Gastric hypersecretion
> - Cholesterol gallstones
> - Hepatic disease
> - Impaired renal function
> - Urinary stone formation
> - Metabolic bone disease

CAUSES OF SHORT BOWEL SYNDROME[9]

Neonates and infants

- Necrotizing enterocolitis
- Congenital anomalies
  - Volvulus neonatorum
  - Intestinal aplasia
  - Aganglionosis
  - Meconium ileus
- Intussusception
- Neoplasia

Adults (in order of frequency)

- Inflammatory bowel disease (Crohn's)
- Mesenteric vascular occlusion
  - Arterial thrombosis or embolism
  - Venous thrombosis
  - Dissecting aortic aneurysm
  - Trauma
  - Intestinal strangulation
- Radiation enteritis
- Midgut volvulus
- Multiple fistula
- Small bowel neoplasia
- Tuberculosis

CAUSES OF MALABSORPTION[9]

- Failure of intraluminal digestion
  - Cholestasis
  - Pancreatic insufficiency
  - Poor mixing
  - Bacterial overgrowth
  - Drugs
- Failure of mucosal absorption
  - Coeliac disease
  - Tropical sprue
  - Whipple's disease
  - Hypogammaglobulinaemia

- Lymphoma, a-chain disease
- Infections
- Radiation damage
- Mesenteric ischaemia
- Enzyme deficiencies – Crohn's disease
- Short bowel syndrome

INFLAMMATORY BOWEL DISEASE

CLINICAL AND PATHOLOGICAL FEATURES OF CROHN'S DISEASE AND ULCERATIVE COLITIS

Clinical features	Crohn's disease	Ulcerative colitis 11 +13
Rectal bleeding	Unusual	Common
Abdominal pain	Common	Unusual
Spontaneous fistula	Sometimes	Very rare never
Mass	Common	Unusual
Perianal infections	30–40%	15%
Rectal involvement	50%	95%

EXTRA GASTROINTESTINAL MANIFESTATIONS OF INFLAMMATORY BOWEL DISEASE (AS PERCENT OF CASES)[13]

	Crohn's	Ulcerative colitis
Eyes		
• Uveitis	4%	4%
• Episcleritis		
• Conjunctivitis		
Joints		
• Monoarticular arthritis	14%	11%
• Ankylosing spondylitis	2–6%	
• Sacroilitis	both 15–18%	
Skin		
• Erythema nodosum	5–10%	2%
• Pyoderma gangrenosum	1%	2%
• Vasculitis		
Liver and biliary tree		
• Fatty change	Common	Common
• Pericholangitis	19%	25%
• Sclerosing cholangitis	<1%	12%
• Chronic active hepatitis	Uncommon	Uncommon
• Cirrhosis	7%	19%
• Cholangiocarcinoma	Uncommon	Uncommon

	Crohn's	Ulcerative colitis
Kidney stones	30%	–
Gallbladder stones	30%	5% (as in normal population)
Pathology		
• Perianal involvement	Common	Less common
• Granulomas	Common	Absent
• Fistula	Common	Uncommon
• Inflammation	Deep (transmural)	Superficial
	Patchy	Continuous
• Goblet cells	Present	Depleted
• Crypt abscesses	+	++(common)

INVESTIGATIONS

Hb, FBC, ESR, U&Es, electrolyte imbalance, LFTs-albumin reduced AXR, barium enema (not performed on toxic patients in case of perforation), sigmoidoscopy, colonoscopy. (In Crohn's disease add folate, vitamin B_{12}, CRP elevated, barium meal and follow through, USS and CT – for abscesses.)

Radiology	Crohn's	Ulcerative colitis
Distribution of disease	Skin lesions	Usually continuous from rectum
Strictures	Often	Rare usually carcinoma
Small bowel involvement	Often, skin lesions	Backwash ileitis
Mucosa	Cobblestones, fissures	Small ulcers, oedema, pseudo polyps
		Deep ulcers

Endoscopy	Crohn's	Ulcerative colitis
Rectal involvement	50%	>95%
Appearance	Oedema, ulcers	Uniform, continuous, granular
	Normal areas friable	

Prognosis		
Medicine	Inadequate in 80%	80% successful
	(50% of patients will require surgery at some point)	
Surgery	Often recurrence	Cure is possible
Risk of cancer	Small	Definite (2% at 10 years, 30% at 30 years)

COMPLICATIONS OF CROHN'S DISEASE[9]

- Dangerous acute complications
  - Perforation, dilation
  - Severs haemorrhage
- Chronic subacute complications
  - Abscess
  - Fistula, e.g. watering can perineum
  - Obstruction
- Malignancy (rare)

TREATMENT OF CROHN'S DISEASE

- Medical
  - 5-Aminosalicylic acid (colitis responds better that small bowel disease)
  - Steroids in acute episodes
  - Azathioprine immunosuppression in severe disease
- Surgical treatment

INDICATIONS FOR SURGERY IN CROHN'S DISEASE

- Recurrent intestinal obstruction
- Bleeding
- Perforation
- Failure of medical therapy
- Intestinal fistula
- Fulminant colitis
- Malignant change (less common than with ulcerative colitis)
- Perianal disease
- Treatment *Aim – to conserve as much bowel as possible:*
  - Stricturoplasty
  - Limited resection
  - Drainage of intra-abdominal abscesses
  - Ileostomy to de-function inflamed bowel
  - Subtotal colectomy with permanent end ileostomy (ileoanal pouches are contra-indicated in Crohn's)

ULCERATIVE COLITIS

Site of ulcerative colitis
- Rectosigmoid only site of inflammation in 60% of cases
- Up to splenic flexure in further 25%
- Total colitis in the remaining 15%

Markers of a severe attack of ulcerative colititis[13]
- Stool frequency – >6 stools/day with blood
- Fever – >37.5°C
- Tachycardia – >90/min
- ESR – >30 mm/h
- Anaemia – Hb <10 g/dl
- Albumin – <30 g/l

LOCAL COMPLICATIONS OF ULCERATIVE COLITIS[5]

- Toxic megacolon
- Colonic perforation
- Massive haemorrhage
- Colonic stricture
- Colonic carcinoma
- Perianal suppuration/disease

TREATMENT OF ULCERATIVE COLITIS

- Anticolitics
  - 5-Aminosalicylic acid (5-ASA)
  - (Salazopyrin SE infertility, olsalazine, enteric-coated mesalazine)
- Steroid preparations (hydrocortisone foam, prednisalone enemas or oral)
- Antidiarrhoeal drugs

INDICATIONS FOR COLECTOMY IN ULCERATIVE COLITIS[5]

- Elective
  - Failure of medical therapy – inadequate control, frequent hospitalization, need for continuous or repeated courses of steroid therapy
  - Prophylactic during cancer surveillance – dysplasia, villous adenomatous change and ectopic colonic mucosa
- Urgent – failure of medical therapy to achieve improvement within 5 days of intensive treatment for a severe attack
- Emergency
  - Toxic megacolon which does not improve within 48–72 h with intensive medical treatment
  - Colonic perforation
  - Massive haemorrhage (very rare indication)
- Types
  - Proctocolectomy and permanent ileostomy (panproctocolectomy)
  - Subtotal colectomy mucous fistula and permanent ileostomy
  - Restorative panproctocolectomy

LOCAL COMPLICATIONS OF A TERMINAL ILEOSTOMY[5]

- Stenosis
- Prolapse
- Peristomal irritation and fistulas
- Para-ileostomy hernia
- Ileostomy diarrhoea
- Prestomal ileitis

SMALL BOWEL FISTULA[5]

- The majority of small bowel fistula (80–90%) follow operations (anastomotic leakage or iatrogenic injury). Modern conservative management results in successful closure in 70–80% but a mortality rate of 6–10%.
- Favourable prognostic factors include:
  - Distal (ileal) fistula
  - Output <500 ml/day (low output fistula)
  - Late occurrence (after 14th postoperative day)
  - Absence of associated fistula
  - No wound dehiscence
- Conservative treatment
  - Nutritional support
  - Meticulous collection of discharge
  - Skin/stoma care
  - Control of sepsis
- Absolute indications for operative intervention are:
  - Distal intestinal obstruction
  - Peritonitis
  - Abscess formation
  - Bowel discontinuity
  - Presence of malignant disease
  - Persistent inflammatory bowel disease

LARGE BOWEL

CAUSES OF CHRONIC INTESTINAL OBSTRUCTION

- Carcinoma of colon or rectum (especially near the rectosigmoid junction)
- Diverticulitis
- Strictures
  - Ischaemic colitis
  - Endometriosis
  - Crohn's disease
- Metastatic deposits(especially in the pelvis from gastric, colonic or genitourinary tumours)
- Hirschsprung's disease (especially in its 'adult' form)
- Idiopathic megacolon
- Pseudo-obstruction
- Anastomotic stenosis (especially after colorectal operations)

CAUSES OF LARGE BOWEL OBSTRUCTION[11]

- Carcinoma of the colon
- Diverticular disease
- Volvulus, usually sigmoid occasionally caecal
- Crohn's disease
- External hernia
- Strictures – radiation, ischaemic, anastomotic, inflammatory

VOLVULUS

Sigmoid volvulus is predisposed to by:[11]
- A long redundant sigmoid colon
- A very high fibre diet
- Chronic constipation and laxative abuse
- Psychiatric and senile disorders

Investigations

AXR 'Coffee bean' arising out of the left pelvis, 'bird's beak' on barium enema

Treatment

Decompression by sigmoidoscopy, flatus tube left *in situ* for 48 h. Laparotomy if there is suspected gangrene or perforation

CAECAL VOLVULUS

Caused by an excessively mobile caecum and ascending colon, a defect in rotation in the caecum retaining its mesentery

Investigation

AXR dilated caecum in left upper quadrant

Treatment

- Laparotomy, untwisting and caecostomy if the bowel is viable. A right hemicolectomy if gangrenous
- A caecal diameter of 15 cm indicates imminent ischaemic necrosis and perforation[11]

Differentiation between viable and non-viable intestine		
Intestine	**Viable**	**Non-viable**
Circulation	Dark colour becomes lighter No bleeding if mesentery is pricked	Dark colour remains Mesentery bleeds if pricked
Peritoneum	Shiny	Dull and lustreless
Intestinal	Firm – pressure rings may or may not persist	Flabby, thin and friable – pressure rings persist; no peristalsis
Musculature	Not disappear	Peristalsis may be observed

DIVERTICULITIS

DIVERTICULAR DISEASE

- Outpouching of colonic mucosa through muscular wall
  - Points of weakness
    - Entry of blood vessels
    - Between longitudinal strips

- Raised intraluminal pressure – muscular incoordination/spasm
- Common, increasing with age, Western world, rare in Africa
- Diet related, low fibre in Western diet
- 5% associated hiatus hernia and gallstones (Saints Triad)
- Mainly sigmoid plus descending colon not rectum (strong muscular wall)

COMPLICATIONS

- Diverticulitis – persistent lower abdominal pain, fever, leucocytosis
- Recurrent diverticulitis
- Pericolic abscess
- Perforation – peritonitis
- Rectal bleeding – haemorrhage
- Fistula formation – colovesical, colovaginal, coloenteric, colocutaneous
- Intestinal obstruction (stricturing from fibrosis)

INVESTIGATIONS

To exclude malignancy and to confirm diagnosis.

- Rigid sigmoidoscopy
- Barium enema or colonoscopy

MANAGEMENT

- Uncomplicated – high fibre diet, bulk laxatives, antispasmodics
- Severe uncomplicated – sigmoid myotomy, colectomy
- Diverticulitis – i.v. fluids, broad spectrum i.v. antibiotics
- Abscess – percutaneous drainage
- Fistula – election resection, primary anastomosis
- Haemorrhage – resuscitation, colectomy (if life threatening)
- Obstruction – possible resection (Hartmann's procedure), possible delayed reanastomosis
- Perforation – laparotomy, peritoneal lavage, antibiotics, possible resection, possible delayed anastomosis

DIFFERENTIATION DIVERTICULITIS FROM CARCINOMA OF THE COLON

	Diverticulitis	Carcinoma
History	Long	Short
Pain	More common	25% painless
Mass	25% have tenderness	
Bleeding persistently	17% often profuse, periodic	65% usually small amounts
Radiograph	Diffuse change	Localized – no relaxation with propantheline bromide
Sigmoidoscopy	Inflammatory change over an area	No inflammation until ulcer is reached
Colonoscopy	No carcinoma seen	Carcinoma seen and biopsied

LARGE BOWEL NEOPLASIA

CLASSIFICATION OF INTESTINAL POLYPS[13]

Type	Solitary	Multiple polyposis syndrome
Hamartomas	Peutz–Jegher Juvenile	Peutz–Jegher syndrome Juvenile polyposis Cronkite–Canada syndrome
Inflammatory	Ulcerative colitis Crohn's colitis Schistosomiasis	Inflammatory polyposis
Neoplastic	Adenoma-tubular tubovillious or villous Carcinoid	Familial adenomatous polyposis
Miscellaneous	Metaplastic (or hyperplastic) Lymphoid	Benign lymphoid polyposis

CHANCE OF MALIGNANT CHANGE RELATED TO POLYP SIZE IN THE COLON OR RECTUM

Size (mm)	Malignant change
<0.5	<1.0%
10–19	5%
20–24	9%
>25	14%

COLORECTAL CARCINOMA

Epidemiology

- 18,000 deaths p.a. M = F
- Second highest cause of cancer deaths in men, third highest cause in women
- Peak incidence is at 60 years of age, but 5% occur <30 years of age
- Site of occurrence (45% rectal, 25% sigmoid, 20% caecum, 10% colon; ascending, transverse, splenic flecture, descending and hepatic flecture in order of frequency)
  - Predominantly Western world disease
  - High fat/protein, low roughage diet
  - Genetic predisposition
    - Chromosome 5
    - Familial adenomatous polyposis
- Spread
  - Local invasion
    - Perforation
    - Pelvic viscera

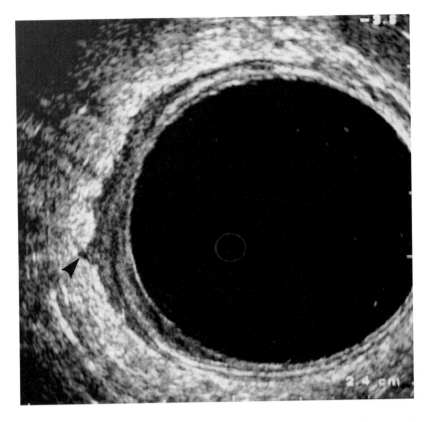

Figure 5.4 Endorectal ultrasound showing advanced rectal cancer with extension into perirectal fat. From: *Fundamentals of Surgical Practice;* Greenwich Medical Media, 1998: page 297.

- Colovesical/vaginal fistula
- Lymph nodes local/distant
- Blood, liver + +, occ lung, brain
- Location – rectum 40%, sigmoid 25%, left colon 15%, caecum 15%

Dukes' staging
- A – tumour confined to bowel wall
- B – serosa breached, no lymph node involvement
- C1 – local lymph nodes involved (mesocolic border)
- C2 – distant nodes involved
- (D) – disseminated disease

CLINICAL FEATURES

Depends on site of lesion:

Left

- Direct effects of lesion
  - Rectal bleeding
  - Change in bowel habit
    - Increased liquid stool or mucus
    - Constipation, tenesmus
  - Obstruction – acute/subacute

Right – systemic effects of malignancy

- Weight loss
- Fatigue, lethargy

Both

- Perforation
- Palpable mass
- Cachexia, anaemia
- Abdominal mass/palpable liver
- Rectal lesion on p.r.
- FBC, U&E, LFT,
- CEA
- Sigmoidoscopy +/– Bx – proceed to urgent barium enema or colonoscopy

TREATMENT

- Curative
  - Excision of lesion with local mesentery and blood supply
  - Pre- or postoperative adjuvant radiotherapy/chemotherapy
- Palliative
  - Surgery for symptomatic relief only
  - General patient care

TYPES OF CURATIVE SURGERY (SEE FIGURE 5.5)

Right-sided lesion	Right or extended right hemicolectomy
Left-sided lesion	Left hemicolectomy*
Sigmoid colon	Sigmoid colectomy*
High rectal lesion	Anterior resection*
Low rectal	Abdominoperineal resection (permanent stoma)

*May be covered with a temporary defunctioning colostomy.

EMERGENCY OR PALLIATIVE SURGERY

Colectomy or Hartmann's procedure or a defunctioning colostomy

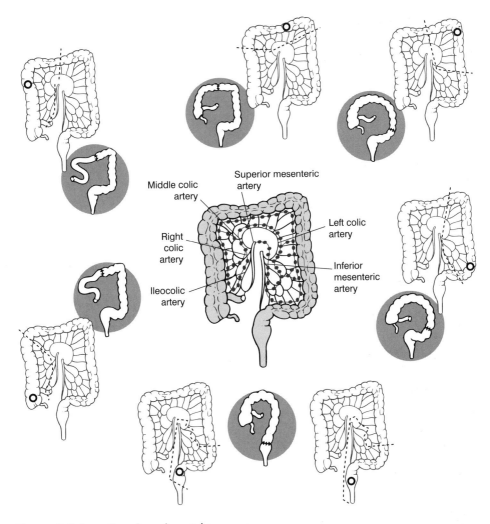

Figure 5.5 Resections for colorectal tumours.

COMPLICATIONS OF SURGERY

General – wound/chest infection; DVT/PE

Specific

- Immediate
  - Bleeding from pelvic vessels
  - Damage to ureters
  - Damage to spleen in left sided mobilization
- Short-term – anastomotic leak
  - Ischaemic cut ends of bowel
  - Infection or haematoma at site of anastomosis
  - Poor general nutritional state of patient

- Long-term
  - Recurrence of disease
  - Stomal or anastomotic stricture
- Adjuvant treatment – clinical trials

PROGNOSIS

- Dependant on stage A – >90% (5YS)
- B – >80%
- C1 – ~ 60%
- C2 – ~ 30%
- D – <5%

FOLLOW UP

- Postcurative treatment
  - 3-monthly clinic appointment
  - 1-year colonoscopy

SCREENING

- At risk individuals – genetic counselling
- General population
  - Mode of screening
    - FOB/CEA/colonoscopy
    - Efficacy of method versus cost and provision of services (Hardcastle trial)

Incidence of malignancy in various gastrointestinal disorders, compared to familial adenomatous polyposis

- Familial adenomatous polyposis (100%)
- Barrett's oesophagus (15%)
- Chronic ulcerative colitis (13%)
- Coeliac disease (13%)
- Pernicious anaemia (<5%)
- Postgastrectomy stomach (<5%)

COMPLICATIONS OF COLOSTOMIES[14]

- Prolapse
- Retraction
- Necrosis of the distal end
- Stenosis of the orifice
- Colostomy hernia
- Bleeding (usually from granulomas around the margin of the colostomy)
- Colostomy 'diarrhoea' – this is usually an infective enteritis and will respond to oral metronidazole 200 mg three times daily

LOWER GASTROINTESTINAL BLEEDING[10,13]

- Bright red blood or blood mixed with stools per rectal
- Exclude upper gastrointestinal causes first

Causes

- Haemorrhoids (common with small recurrent bleeds)
- Anal fissure (common)
- Colitis usually associated with diarrhoea
  - Crohn's
  - Ulcerative
  - Infective
  - Ischaemic (less common)
- Carcinoma (colorectal and anal)
- Polyps (small frequent bleeds)
- Carcinoma of the caecum (often occult)
- Diverticular (uncommon)
- Meckel's diverticulum
- Solitary ulcer of the rectum
- Angiodysplasia (occult and rare)
- Irradiation colitis or proctitis
- Rectal prolapse
- Mesenteric infarction
- Aorto-enteric fistula
- Massive upper gastrointestinal haemorrhage
- Trauma
- Bleeding diathesis

Management

Mainly conservative

- Full examination including p.r. + sigmoidoscopy
- Resuscitate as above
- Monitor
- Most bleeding settles within 48 h with no action, then semiurgent colonoscopy or barium enema

Continued bleeding

- More than eight units transfused
- Patient remains unstable
- Evidence of active bleeding

Investigations possible

- Mesenteric angiography (if available and possible)

Treatment

- Laparotomy requiring colectomy plus examination for bleeding point
- Right hemicolectomy or Hartmann's as appropriate

ANORECTAL CONDITIONS

DISORDERS OF THE ANORECTAL MUSCULATURE[5]

- Rectal prolapse
  - Complete
  - Partial
- Solitary rectal ulcer
- Anal incontinence
  - Idiopathic
  - Descending perineum syndrome
  - Pelvic floor neuropathy

FACTORS MAINTAINING ANAL CONTINENCE:

- Anal sphincters
  - Internal (IAS) – PNS is inhibitory and SNS is stimulatory
  - External (EAS) – voluntary striated muscle innervated by the pudendal nerve
- Puborectalis and the anorectal angle – striated muscle innervated by the pudendal nerve
- Intact rectal and anal sensation – the sensation of filling produces an additional reflex factor in continence
- Others factors
  - The nature of the rectal reservoir (size and compliance)
  - Formation of bulky and solid faeces

Origins of anal incontinence[8]

- Descent	- Damage
- Perineal descent	- Wounds
- Prolapsing haemorrhoid	- Surgical procedures
- Rectal prolapse	- Childbirth
- Destruction	- Denervation
- Malignant tumours	- Spinal injuries
- Irradiation	- Neurosurgical procedures
- Debility	- Spina bifida
- Illness	- Demented
- Old age	- Senility
- Deficiency – congenital abnormalities	- Psychological abnormality

---

ANORECTAL INVESTIGATIONS

- Anal manometry
- Rectal sensation
- Electromyography
- Endoanal ultrasound
- Defecating proctography
- Colonic transit time

Causes of pericoccygeal swellings[12]
- Pilonidal sinus
- Postanal dermoid cyst
- Chordoma
- Sacrococcygeal teratoma

ANAL CANAL DISORDERS

- Anal canal = rectum from level of pelvic brim to anal verge

Common disorders
- Anorectal sepsis
  - Abscess
  - Fistula *in ano*
- Anal fissure
- Pilonidal sinus/abscess
- Haemorrhoids

ANORECTAL ABSCESS

- Infection of anal gland (90%); extension of a cutaneous lesion
  - *Escherichia coli*, bacteroides, *Staphylococcus aureus*, *Streptococcus* may reflect aetiology (i.e. bowel versus skin origin)
- Associated conditions:
  - Diabetes, immunosuppression
  - Abdominal sepsis (Crohn's)
  - Existing fistula *in ano*
  - Painful or erythematous fluctuant swelling in perianal region
    - Perianal (60%)
    - Ischiorectal (30%)
    - Submucous (5%)
    - Pelvirectal between levator ani and pelvic peritoneum

Treatment
- Incision and drainage of collection (urgent), packing of cavity
- Healing in 2–6 weeks if no underlying pathology
- Failure to resolve or recurrence then investigate for cause

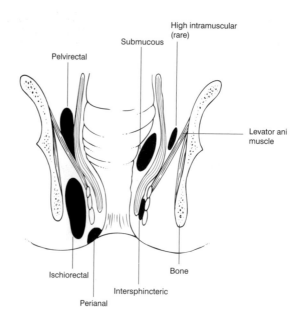

Figure 5.6 Sites of anal abscesses.

FISTULA *IN ANO*

Definition – granulation tissue line tract linking perianal skin to anorectal canal
- Low-opening below anorectal ring
- High-opening above anorectal ring

Aetiology
- Recurrent or incompletely resolved sepsis
- Crohn's' disease
- (TB)

Symptoms
- Persistent perianal discharge
- Pain if opening blocked

Investigation
- External opening visible or palpable on examination/proctoscopy
- Injection with hydrogen peroxide may demonstrate internal opening
- MRI
- Goodsall's rule – external opening
  - *anterior* = direct tract
  - *posterior* = horseshoe tract

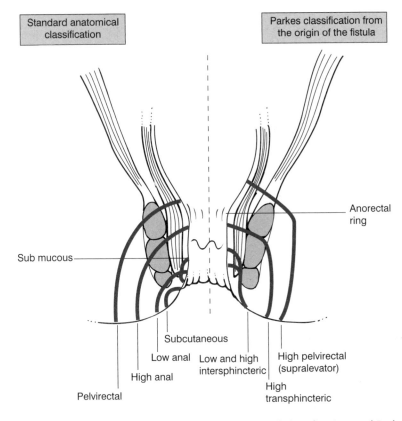

Figure 5.7 Types of anorectal fistula. Standard anatomical classification and Parkes' classification from the origin of the fistula.

Treatment

- Low – tract may be probed and laid open to allow secondary healing
- High
  - Above procedure will result in incontinence
  - Specialist centre referral
  - Staged procedure with possible defunctioning colostomy

ANAL FISSURE

Definition – longitudinal mucosal ulcer in lower anal canal. 90% is posterior midline

Aetiology

- Constipation – hard stool and straining
- Trauma
- Posthaemorrhoidectomy
- Crohn's disease
- Symptoms – pain on defecation with bleeding or discharge

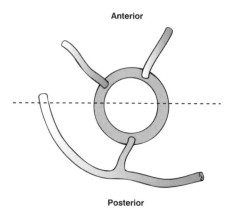

Anterior

Posterior

Figure 5.8 Goodsall's rule relating to anal fistula. If the external opening of the fistula is in the anterior half of the anus, the fistula should have a relatively direct track, whereas if the external opening is in the posterior half, the fistula may have multiple openings and should form a connection to a single internal orifice (usually midline). It is possible for the fistula to extend laterally on both sides leading to a horseshoe fistula.

Investigations

- EUA/proctoscopy
- Conservative, dietary advice/laxatives

TREATMENT OF ANAL FISSURES[28]

- Conservative – stool softeners, analgesic jelly and GTN – heals acute fissures in 50%
- Surgical
  - Manual dilatation of the anus (MDA) – leads to temporary postoperative soiling in 39% (falling out of favour)
  - Sphincterotomy – lateral – heals 96% of patients within 3 weeks
  - Posterior – leads to disturbances of continence in 25%

PILONIDAL SINUS (A NEST OF HAIRS)

- Blind granulation tissue lined tract in natal cleft
- Possible formation following epidermal overgrowth of hair/hair follicle
- More common in hairy men, long distance drivers
- Intermittent infection
  - Purulent discharge
  - Pain
  - Abscess formation

  may;

  - Resolve spontaneously
  - Resolve following course of antibiotics
  - Abscess formation requires incision and drainage

- Recurrent inflammation
- Non-resolving discharge

Treatment
- Wide local excision of sinus
- Marsupialization of tract

HAEMORRHOIDS

A common problem
- F>M
- Pregnancy, obese
- Dilatation of rectal venous plexus 'cushions'
- Grades
  I – within anal canal
  II – prolapsing but spontaneously reducible
  III – prolapsed, requires manual relocation
  IV – prolapse permanent
- Bright red rectal bleeding
- Pain if large or prolapsed or thrombosed

Treatment

Aim – treat symptoms not haemorrhoids
- Advise high fibre diet (reduces strain on defecation)
- Course of up to 3 × injections with oily phenol (a sclerosant)
  - Reduces bleeding and may shrink size
  - Banding rubber band ligation of pedicle
- Formal haemorrhoidectomy – risk of incontinence, anal stenosis, anal fissure formation

CAUSES OF PRURITUS ANI[12]
- Mucous discharge from the anus caused by:
  - Haemorrhoids
  - Polyps
  - Skin tags
  - Condylomata
  - Fissure
  - Fistula
  - Carcinoma of the anus
- Vaginal discharge caused by
  - Trichomonas vaginitis
  - Monilial vaginitis
  - Cervicitis
  - Gonorrhoea
- Skin diseases
  - Tinea cruris
  - Fungal infections especially monilial infections in diabetics

- Parasites – threadworms
- Faecal soiling
  - Poor hygiene
  - Incontinence
  - Diarrhoea
- Psychoneuroses

Treatment

- Hygienic measures
- Hydrocortisone – only in cases with dermatitis
- Strapping the buttocks apart

ABDOMINAL WALL HERNIA

CAUSES OF ABDOMINAL HERNIA[12]

- An anatomical weakness
  - Structures pass through an abdominal wall
  - Muscles fail to overlap
  - No musculature only scar tissue (e.g. umbilicus)
- An acquired weakness following trauma
- High intra-abdominal pressure from coughing, straining, abdominal distension

CHARACTERISTICS OF INGUINAL HERNIA

Infant

- Present in 2% of live born babies (4% in male)
- Male-to-female predominance 9:1
- 60% of children with inguinal hernia present with incarceration, but they rarely progress to strangulation

Adult

- 5–10% of males are affected
- 10:1 male-to-female predominance
- 60% are direct, 35% indirect, 10% combined
- 80,000 hernia repairs are performed annually, 10% for recurrence
- Annual probability of strangulation is 0.3–3%
- Indirect hernias are 10 times as likely to strangulate
- Mortality of strangulated inguinal hernias is 7–14%

Note: the mortality rate *n* strangulated hernias increases with age – 3% at 60 years, 6% at 70 years, 12% at 80 years.

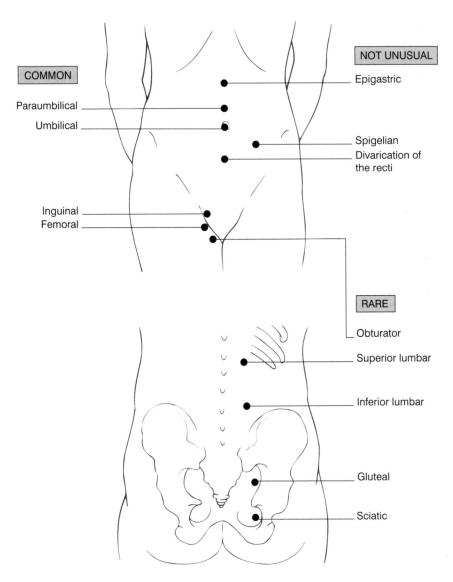

COMMON

NOT UNUSUAL

Paraumbilical

Umbilical

Epigastric

Spigelian

Divarication of
the recti

Inguinal

Femoral

RARE

Obturator

Superior lumbar

Inferior lumbar

Gluteal

Sciatic

Figure 5.9 Sites of external hernia.

> **Royal College of Surgeons of England Clinical Guidelines on Management of Groin Hernias in Adults**
>
> - Indirect and symptomatic direct hernias should be repaired to relieve symptoms and eliminate the small long-term risk of strangulation
> - Easily reducible direct hernias need not necessarily be repaired but should be reviewed within 1 year
> - Recurrent inguinal hernia should be managed as above
> - Irreducible or newly presenting inguinal hernias should be repaired promptly to avoid strangulation

PRINCIPLES OF EMERGENCY HERNIA MANAGEMENT

- Patient must be resuscitated
- Hernia reduced
- Defect repaired

Structures which form the spermatic cord[5]

Three arteries	Three nerves	Three structures
Testicular	Ilio-inguinal	Pampiniform plexus
Cremasteric	Genital branch of the genitofemoral	Vas deferens
Vas deferens	Sympathetic	Remnants of the processus vaginalis

CHARACTERISTICS OF FEMORAL HERNIA

- More common in women than men (F:M = 2.5:1)
- Account for 11% of all groin hernia and 35–50% of all strangulated hernia
- Are equally common as indirect inguinal hernia in women
- 50% present with strangulation; have double the bowel resection rate of inguinal hernia and carry a 3–15% mortality rate
- Probability of strangulation at 1 month after diagnosis is 22%, and at 21 months it is 45%

THREE APPROACHES TO THE FEMORAL HERNIA

- Abdominal, suprapubic, retroperitoneal, preperitoneal or extraperitoneal (eponyms Cheatle, Hemnry, McEvedy)
- Inguinal or high (Annandale, Lothiessen or Moscowitz)
- Crural or low (Bassini, Lockwood)

SITES OF INTERNAL HERNIAS

- Foramen of Winslow (the portal vein, common bile duct, and hepatic artery lie in its free border)
- A hole in the mesentery

- A hole in the transverse mesocolon
- A defect in the broad ligament
- Congenital or acquired diaphragmatic hernia
- One of the retroperitoneal fossa, of which those about the duodenum and caecum and appendix are most important
  - Fossae about the duodenum:
    - Left paraduodenal fossa – the inferior mesenteric vein lies in its free border
    - Right duodeno-jejunal fossa – the superior mesenteric artery runs in its free border
  - Fossae about the caecum and appendix:
    - Superior ileocaecal fossa – between the general mesentery and a fold of peritoneum raised by the anterior caecal branch of the ileocolic artery
    - Inferior ileocaecal fossa – between the 'bloodless' fold of Treves and the mesentery of the appendix
    - The retrocaecal fossa behind the caecum
  - Intersigmoid fossa is situated in the base of the pelvic mesocolon

CAUSES OF AN INCISIONAL HERNIA[6]

- Technical factors
  - Postoperative haematoma, necrosis and sepsis
  - Inept closure – using absorbable sutures on aponeurosis, too small bites and knot failure
  - Placing drains or stomas in the wound
  - Inappropriate incision
- Tissue factors
  - Age
  - Immunosuppression, diabetes, jaundice and renal failure
  - Obesity
  - Malignant disease

6

VASCULAR SYSTEM

TYPES OF ARTERIAL DISEASE

- Atherosclerosis
- Embolic
- Aneurysm
- Arteritis
- Infective
- Vasospastic
- Neoplastic

ATHEROSCLEROSIS

- Hardening of vessel wall
- Narrowing of lumen
- Focal intimal accumulation of lipids and fibrous tissue formin a plaque
  - Activated macrophage infiltration
  - Smooth muscle proliferation
- Calcification

Risk factors

- Smoking
- Hyperlipidaemia
- diabetes
- Hypertension

Clinical features

- Chronic
- Acute on chronic
  - Onset of symptoms
- Location of lesion(s)
  - Disease may be present at multiple levels
  - Collateral circulation alters severity of disease

Investigations

- Doppler probe
  - Presence of vessel pulse signals
  - Ankle-brachial pressure index – approximation of severity of vascular impairment
- Duplex Scan
- Arteriography
- MRA
  - Anatomical location and extent of lesions
  - Plan for further intervention

CAROTID DISEASE

- Lesion at bifurcation of common carotid artery and internal carotid artery (see Figure 6.2)
- Stenosis and site for formation of platelet emboli
  - Transient ischaemic attacks
  - Amaurosis fugax
  - Cerebral infarction

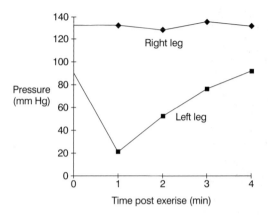

Figure 6.1 Exercise test result showing a normal pressure response in the right leg and an abnormal response (the pressure drops suddenly on exercise as perfusion is inadequate to meet demand) in the left where there is femoropopliteal occlusion. From *Fundamentals of Surgical Practice*; Greenwich Medical Media, 1998: page 307.

- Without surgery >5%/year chance of CVA
- >75% stenosis and symptomatic suggests indication for surgery
- <75% stenosis or asymptomatic, no benefit over medical management

SURGICAL TREATMENT

Carotid endarterectomy
- 1% mortality
- 1% CVA risk
- Hypoglossal nerve at risk in dissection

SUBCLAVIAN ARTERY

- Proximal subclavian artery stenosis
  - 'Steal syndrome' – blood diverted down vertebral a when ipsilateral upper limb inuse
  - Symptoms of verto-basilar insufficiency
  - vertigo, tinnitus, nausea, collapse
- Surgery – endarterectomy or jump graft

SUPERIOR MESENTERIC AND INFERIOR MESENTERIC ARTERIES

- Stenosis – abdominal pain, weight loss, diarrhoea
- Occlusion – mesenteric infarction
- Surgery – endarterectomy or bypass
- Bowel resection of non-viable gut in acute situation

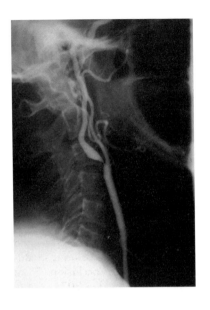

Figure 6.2 Internal carotid artery stenosis. From *Fundamentals of Surgical Practice*; Greenwich Medical Media, 1998: page 312.

RENAL ARTERY

- Stenosis
  - Decreased renal blood flow
  - Activation of renin–angiotensin–aldosterone system
  - Hypertension

Treatment
- Transluminal angioplasty/endarterectomy

AORTO-ILIAC DISEASE

- Stenotic lesions at distal aorta/proximal common iliac artery
- Collateral vessels available, symptoms masked
- Chronic
  - Buttock pain, upper thigh pain
  - Impotence (Lehriche syndrome)
- Acute – bilateral acutely ischaemic limbs (saddle embolus)

Treatment
- Surgery
  - Transluminal angioplasty
  - Discrete, localized lesions
  - 50–60% 5-year patency
- Aorto-bifemoral graft
  - Dacron = 90% 5-year patency
  - mortality rate = 5%
- Unfit/high-risk patients
  - Axillo-bifemoral
  - Femoral–femoral crossover graft – <60% 5-year patency
- Complications – see AAA repair

FEMORAL ARTERY AND DISTAL DISEASE

- Stenotic lesion mainly in superior femoral artery (adductor canal)
- Multiple distal lesion may occur
- Chronic
  - Claudication – progressive
  - Skin changes (atrophic)
- Critical
  - Rest pain +/– ulceration/gangrene
  - Ankle systolic pressure <50 mmHg (non-diabetic); <30 mmHg diabetic
- Acute – pale, pulseless, parasthesia, paresis, cold (embolic usually)

Treatment

- Surgery
  - Transluminal angioplasty
  - If Discrete single lesion <10 cm length
  - 40–50% 5-year patency

All patients

- Additional conservative management
  - Stop smoking
  - Control diet/lipids/diabetes
  - Exercise

	5–year patency	
	Vein graft	**Prosthetic graft**
Femoro-popliteal	65–70%	55–65%
Femoro-distal bypass	50%	20–30%

Failed graft and recurrent critical ischaemia may result in amputation.

Ankle brachial pressures index (ABPI)

The pressure at the ankle should be the same of higher the brachial pressure (index 0.9-1.2). Rigid atherosclerotic arteries in diabetics may give spurious high pressures at the ankle. An index of 0.7 indicates moderate ischaemia and if below 0.5 is usually associated with rest pain and severe ischaemia.

Exercise testing

Some patients with occlusive disease will have normal ankle resting pressure whereas on exercise on a treadmill, the pressure will fall. In a normal patient it will rise due to increased systolic pressure and peripheral vasodilation

Graft complications

- Anastomotic leak
- Thrombosis and occlusion
- Infection

Future developments

- Evaluation of endovascular prosthetic stents

AMPUTATIONS OF LOWER LIMB

Indications

- Chronic critical or acute ischaemia
  - Atherosclerosis
  - Buerger's disease
  - Embolism
- Infection
  - Gangrene
  - Uncontrollable sepsis
- Malignancy – primary or secondary
- Trauma – non-viable deformity
- Level of amputation
  - Above level of disease, Viable tissue at this level
  - No disease or deformity above
  - Suitable for possible future prosthesis
    - Preservation of knee joint > faster rehabilitation
- Below-knee amputation
  - Minimum of 8 cm tibia below knee required to fit prosthesis
  - Long posterior flap (Burgess amputation)
  - Myoplastic skew flap amputation
- Above-knee amputation – minimum 11 cm above the knee joint required for a functioning prosthesis

EMBOLIC DISEASE

Passage of material within the vascular lumen, resulting in occlusion and obstruction

- Platelet/fibrin aggregates
- Fat
- Air
- Amniotic fluid
- Infective
- Metastatic

Sources of emboli

- Heart
  - Atrial fibrillation
  - Post-myocardial infarction
  - Endocarditis
  - Ventricular aneurysm
  - Mitral valve
  - Prosthetic valve
- Aorta – aneurysm

Site of occlusion

- Points of division
  - Aortic bifurcation (saddle embolus)
  - Popliteal trifurcation – causing ischaemic foot

Symptoms

- Sudden onset of acute ischaemic symptoms
- Pale/pulseless/pain/parasthesia/paresis
- Limb viability diminishes after 4–6 h > irreversible necrosis

Treatment

- Acute embolic event
  - Embolectomy – Fogarty balloon catheter
  - Heparinization postoperatively
  - Overall mortality rate 10–20%
- Acute on chronic event (*in-situ* thrombosis)
- Pre-existing atherosclerosis
- Slower onset of symptoms
  - Consider thrombolytic therapy
  - Under evaluation

THROMBOLYTIC THERAPY

Is a technique whereby the natural thrombolytic activity of the body is stimulated by an activator.

The agents used are:

- Streptokinase (derived from streptococcoi): antigenic, least expensive and effective
- Urokinase (from human urine)
- Tissue plasminogen activator (TPA) non antigenic, most effective and expensive

They may be given as a single bolus (in MI) or as a continuous, pulsed or high dose short term intra-arterial infusion. These activate plasminogen in the thrombus and enhance the normal thrombolytic activity

Indications for use

- Acute thrombus of an artery or bypass graft
- Acute embolism
- Acute thrombosis as a complication of angioplasty
- Thrombosis of a popliteal aneurysm

Contraindications are:

- Critical ischaemia with neurological deficit
- Irreversible ischaemic change
- The early postoperative period

Favourable factors for treatment

- <1 week duration
- Emboli
- Occlusion<10cm

Unfavourable factors

- <1 week duration
- Thrombosis
- Occlusion>10cm

ANEURYSMAL DISEASE

- Definition of aneurysm: a localized, permanent dilation of vascular structure
- True-aneurysm consists of all layers of vessel wall
- False-aneurysm consists of partial thickness of vessel wall only

- Fusiform – along axis of vessel
- Saccular – tangential to axis
- Dissecting-stripping of intima from wall

Causes

Decreased wall strength and/or rise in intraluminal pressure.

Congenital
- Berry aneurysm
- Marfans' syndrome
- Ehlers–Danlos

Acquired
- Trauma/iatrogenic
  - Instrumentation (arterial monitoring lines)
  - Intravenous drug abusers
- Inflammation/infection
  - Syphilis, TB
  - Mycotic
  - Retroperitoneal fibrosis
- Degeneration – atherosclerosis

Common sites

- Aorta – 95% atherosclerosis, 95% below renal
- Iliacs, femoral, popliteal
- Circle of Willis
- Splenic/hepatic/mesenteric (<1%)

Natural history

- Rupture
- Thrombosis
- Local pressure symptoms
- Source of emboli

ABDOMINAL AORTIC ANEURYSM

- Size and symptoms important
- Measured by Ultrasound and CT scan
  - Maximal diameter
  - Length, infra- or suprarenal; involvement of iliacs

Clinical features

- Age >60 years
- M>F
- Previous history or risk factors for atherosclerosis
- Acute

- Rupture
  - Sudden onset acute abdominal/back/buttock pain
  - Collapse
  - Hypovolaemic shock
  - Pulsatile abdominal mass may be felt
- Chronic
  - Vague back/abdominal pain
  - Pulsatile abdominal mass

Differential Diagnosis

- MI
- Peptic ulcer disease
- Pancreatitis
- Renal colic

Management

Acute rupture

- Resuscitation and assessment
  - Is patient otherwise fit to undergo major surgery?
  - No – severe IHD/COAD/advanced malignancy
  - No – conservative management only >100% mortality rate
  - Yes – emergency laparotomy; repair 50% mortality rate + morbidity

Chronic

- For elective repair? – mortality rate of 5% versus risk of spontaneous rupture and death 50% mortality rate
- Diameter >5.5 cm or symptomatic – 12% p.a. risk of rupture – increasing symptoms] rupture may be imminent
- Diameter <5.5 cm
  - Monitor if asymtomatic (0.5%/year risk rupture)
  - Regular USS/CT
  - Consider surgery if
    - >5.5 cm
    - Rapid increase in size
    - Patient increasingly symptomatic

Complications

Early

- Death
  - Hypovolaemic shock
  - Cardiogenic shock
  - ARDS
  - DIC
- Anastomotic leak – haemorrhage
- Reperfusion injury
  - Systemic hyperkalaemia
  - Myoglobinuria – causing renal failure/cardiac arrhythmia
- Acute ischaemia

- Lower limbs; embolectomy may be required
- IMA/SMA disruption; gut ischaemia
- Renal hypoperfusion; renal failure
- Spinal; paraplegia

Late

- Graft
  - Thrombosis
  - Infection
  - Aorto-enteric fistula
  - Sexual dysfunction

Overall 5 YS – 80% post-successful repair

Advances

- Endovascular stenting of small aneurysm – benefits/risks/long-term complications to be evaluated
- Screening
  - Benefit of USS to asymptomatic patients
    - Monitor small aneurysm (small aneurysm study)
    - Consider elective surgery on >5.5 cm
    - No national screening programme yet organized
  - Cost – may not improve mortality/morbidity rates in a screened population as most patients are >70 years of age

VASCULITIDES

Inflammatory changes in arterial wall resulting in swelling; obstruction; ischaemia

Thromboangitis obliterans (Buerger's disease)

- Affects male smokers 20–30 years of age
- Prevalent in India, Asia, Israel
- Results in progressive obliteration of distal medium sized art > progressive obliteration
- Chronic and acute ischaemic changes – gangrene

Antibodies to elastin, type I and II collagen

- Link with HLA A9, B5

Treatment

- Stop smoking
- Steroid +/– anticoagulants
- Sympathectomy or amputation

Takayasu's disease

- Affects females 15–45 years of age; oriental more common
- Rare occlusive disorder of the aorta and brachiocephalic branches
- May cause MI, renal hypertension and bowel ischaemia

Treatment

- Steroid +/– surgical replacement

Giant cell arteritis

- Any part of arterial tree, especially head and neck
- >50 years + F>M
- Northern Europe
- Headache, tender supf tempart noted
- Risk of blindness in ophthalmic a involvement

Treatment

- Biopsy + high dose steroids

Small vessels vasculitides

- Polyarteritis nodosa
- Kawasaki disease
- Wegener's granulomatosis
- Churg–Strauss syndrome
- Henoch–Schoenlein purpura

Treatment

- Mostly medical treatment

Infective arteritis

- TB
- Syphilis
- Leprosy
- Bacterial infections
- Viral infections
- Causes thrombosis, fibrosis, occlusion, aneurysm formation

VASOSPASTIC DISEASE

Vasomotor malfunction of sympathetic supply to small vessels

Raynauds

- Intermittent digital vasospasm without primary cause
  - Local ischaemia gangene
  - Exacerbated by cold, emotion, drugs (OCP, β-blockers), smoking
  - May occur in association with
    - SLE
    - Systemic sclerosis (CREST)
    - PAN
    - Rheumatoid arthritis
    - Sjögren's
- F>M
- Young, bilateral
- Exclude major vessel disease
- Treat conservatively
  - Remove drugs, stop smoking
  - Prostacyclin if gangrene risk
- Poor results from sympathectomy (30–40% recurrence rate)

VASCULAR NEOPLASIA

- Rare
- Carotid body tumour (chemodectoma)
- Angiosarcoma – rapid metastases
- Kaposi sarcoma – AIDS patients
- Glomus tumours

VARICOSE VEINS

Dilatation of superficial veins of lower limbs

Cause

- Primary
  - Genetic
  - Weak vessel structure deficiency of muscle/collagen
    - Incompetence of valve system
    - Retrograde flow from deep system via perforating vessels
    - Increased intramural pressure
    - Progressive dilatation of veins
    - Further incompetence
  - Exacerbating factors
    - Pregnancy
    - Obesity
    - Long periods of standing
- Secondary
  - Post-thrombosis deep system
  - Pelvic tumours
  - Congenital abnormality – Klippel–Trenauny > av fistulas

Clinical presentations

- Non-aesthetic changes in lower limb image
- Bleeding
- Pain
- Ulceration
- Varicose eczema
- Thrombophlebitis, lipodermatosclerosis

Examination

- Trendelenburg tests
- Confirms level of incompetence

LONG SAPHENOUS VEIN (LSV)

- Sapheno-femoral junction incompetence in (90%) of cases
- Mid-thigh/mid-calf perforators
- Distribution of varicosities
- Antero-medial calf/lower thigh
- Medial malleolus

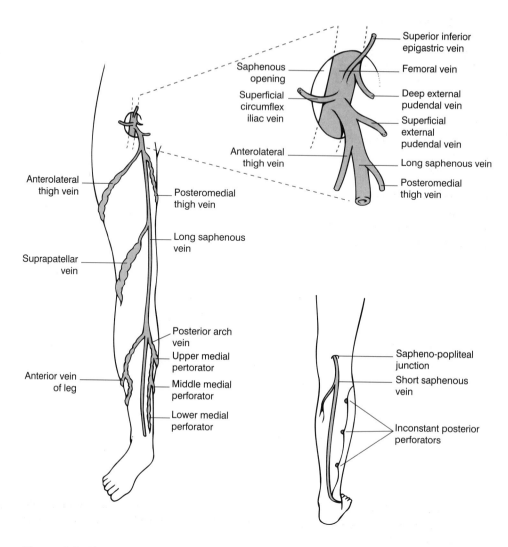

Figure 6.3 The main tributaries of the long and short saphenous and distribution of the perforating veins.

SHORT SAPHENOUS VEIN (SSV)

- Sapheno-popliteal junction
- Mid-calf perforators
- Distribution of varicosities
- Postero-lateral calf
- Popliteal fossa and lateral malleolus

Note: clinical examination can be misleading as to exact nature of problem.

Investigations

- Deep system
- LSV or SSV problem
- Level of incompetence
  - Duplex scan
  - Venography

Indications for surgery

- Cosmetic/patient request (90%)
- Bleeding
- Ulceration

Contra-indications

- 'Pain'
- Deep vein insufficiency (DVI) or previous DVT
- Possible candidate for arterial/cardiac surgery

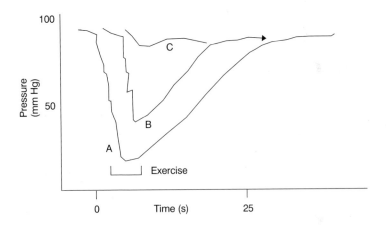

Figure 6.4 Ambulatory pressure measurements. A = normal, B = familial abnormality, C = perforator incompetence. From: *Fundamentals of Surgical Practice*; Greenwich Medical Media, 1998: page 321.

Surgery

LSV

- High tie (SFJ) + strip of LSV + avulsion of varicosities
  - Groin incision
    - SFJ and branches identified and tied
    - Vein stripped to knee level

SSV

- Ligate SPJ + multiple avulsion of varicosities – SPJ best located preoperatively on duplex scan

Complications

- Postoperative bleeding
- Wound infection
- Damage to
  - Saphenous n. – abnormal sensation medial calf
  - Lateral popliteal n. – foot drop
- Recurrence
  - Incomplete isolation of venous system in first operation
  - Incompetence of other system
  - New perforator
  - Deep system incompetence
- Many alternative/private solutions to vvs available, e.g. sclerotherapy
  - Dubious benefit
  - Not available/practised NHS

LEG ULCERS

- 500,000 sufferers in the UK; 1/5 active, F>M

Causes (see Figure 6.5)

- Venous disease
- Arterial disease
- Mixed venous arterial disease
- Neuropathic – diabetes
- Neoplastic
  - SCC – Marjolin's ulcer
  - BCC
  - MM

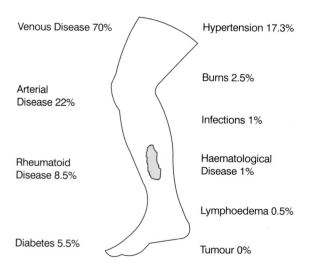

Venous Disease 70%

Hypertension 17.3%

Arterial
Disease 22%

Burns 2.5%

Infections 1%

Rheumatoid
Disease 8.5%

Haematological
Disease 1%

Lymphoedema 0.5%

Diabetes 5.5%

Tumour 0%

Figure 6.5 Conditions associated with leg ulceration. From: *Fundamentals of Surgical Practice*; Greenwich Medical Media, 1998: page 321.

- Chronic other
  - Trauma
    - Pretibial
    - Foreign body
  - Infection – underlying osteomyelitis
  - Inflammation – autoimmune disease

VENOUS ULCERS

- Chronic venous insufficiency of lower limbs
- Fibrin cuff theory
  - Mechanical obstruction to oxygen diffusion
  - Cellular hypoxia
  - Damage results in poor repair
- Oxygen-free radicals theory
  - Released in chronic venous insufficiency
  - Local tissue damage

Clinical features

- Large non-healing ulcers
  - Lower tibia especially medial malleolus
  - Extensive/circumferential
  - May undergo metaplasia and become SCC
- Past history – deep venous insufficiency
- Varicose superficial veins
- Immobility, depression, etc.

Investigations

- Duplex scan
  - Competence of deep and superficial systems
  - Exclude arterial disease

Management

- Conservative
  - 'Four layer' compression bandage
  - Daily dressings
- Surgery – consider split skin grafting to aid rapid healing

No deep vein insufficiency

- Ulcer may heal after treatment of superficial veins

DIABETIC ULCERS

- Arterial insufficiency
  - Macro vessel disease – reduced distal blood flow to limb
  - Micro vessel disease – loss of regulatory function
- Neuropathy
  - Decreased afferent sensation – increased risk of accidental trauma
  - Sympathetic dysfunction – dry skin and so increased damage following trauma
- General – high-risk/poor response to infection

Management of the diabetic foot

- Conservative
  - Control diabetes
  - Regular inspection and chiropody
  - Good-fitting shoes
- Other
  - Treat infections aggressively
  - Improve distal circulation

LYMPHOEDEMA

Accumulation of fluid in extracellular/extravascular fluid compartment – subcutaneous tissues in limbs

Congenital (primary) lymphoedema

- Milroy's disease
  - Lymphoedema congenita – present at birth
  - Lymphoedema praecox – puberty onset
  - Lymphoedema tarda – adult onset
- Non-pitting oedema of lower limbs without other cause
- Hypoplasia of lymphatics
  - Reduced lymphatic vessels in lower limb
  - Demonstrated by lymphangiography
  - Distal lymphatics may 'die off' causing further deterioration – retrograde obliteration
- Varicose lymphatics
  - Dilated tortuous lymph vessels
  - May have congenital av fistula associated

Acquired (secondary) lymphoedema

- Obstruction of main lymphatic vessels, backflow into subcutaneous vessels
- Exclude other systemic causes
  - Hypoproteinaemia
  - Cardiac failure
  - Deep vein thrombosis
- Trauma – major limb trauma
- Iatrogenic
  - Surgical bloc dissection of nodal area, e.g. upper limb oedema post breast surgery
  - Radiotherapy to lymphatic bed
- Infection
  - Repeated acute infections (e.g. barefoot)
  - Chronic bacterial infection, TB, fungus
  - Parasitic – filariasis > elephantiasis
- Malignancy – carcinomatosis

Complications

- Recurrent cellulitis
- Ulceration
- Malignancy (rare) – lymphangiosarcoma (Stewart–Treves syndrome), BCC, SCC, melanoma, fibrous histiocytoma

Management

- Conservative
  - Treat cause (if known)
  - Bed rest
  - Elevation
  - Compression stockings
  - Intermittent limb compression pump
- Surgical
  - Poor results
  - Only in severe debilitating conditions – excision of excess tissue plus reconstruction
  - Deeper/spreading sepsis

THORACIC OUTLET COMPRESSION SYNDROME (TOCS)

Neurological/vascular symptoms

- Proximal compression of
  - Subclavian artery
  - Subclavian vein
  - Brachial plexus T1/C8 roots
- Structures pass over first rib from thorax to upper limb
- Compression by clavicle, scaleus muscles
  - +/– Fibromuscular bands
  - Cervical ribs

Symptoms

Arterial

- Cold, pale (ischaemic)
- Emboli
- 'Raynauds'

Venous

- Cyanosis
- Oedema
- Thrombosis

Nerve

- Pain
- Parasthesia
- Headaches
- Weakness

Differential diagnosis

- C-spine pathology

- Distal nerve compression
- Axilla/chest wall radiation
- Pancoasts tumour
- 'Raynauds'
- Atrial fibrillation (AF) (emboli)
- Clotting disorder leading to > hypercoagulable states (protein C, S deficiency)

Investigations

- CXR
- MRI
- Angiogram

Surgery

- Thoracic outlet decompression may be considered

7

ENDOCRINE SYSTEM

BREAST DISEASE
THYROID
PARATHYROID DISEASE
ADRENAL GLAND DISEASE

BREAST DISEASE

BREAST CANCER

- 20,000 cases per year UK
- 12,000 deaths per year UK
- 1/12–14 overall risk per UK women
- Rare <20 years, increasing risk > 50 years
- West/UK high incidence; low incidence in Japan and Far East
- 1–2% of cases occur in males

High risk groups for breast cancer
- Age >45 years
- Carcinoma of the contralateral breast
- Family history of breast cancer in first-degree relatives
- Nulliparity
- First-term pregnancy >30 years of age
- Early menarche and late natural menopause
- Early artificial menopause
- Previous fibrocystic disease especially in those with proliferative epithelial changes and cellular atypia
- High levels of dietary fat

Pathology

- Invasive
  - Ductal (80–90%)
  - Lobular (5–10%)
  - Paget's (1–2%)

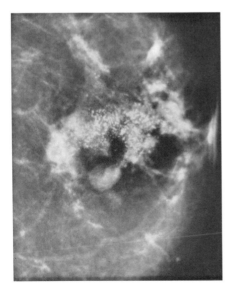

Figure 7.1 Characteristic mammographic appearance of microcalcifications associated with malignancy. From: *Fundamentals of Surgical Practice;* Greenwich Medical Media, 1998: page 356

- *In-situ*
  - Ductal carcinoma *in situ* – 30–50% risk of malignant transformation
  - Lobular carcinoma *in situ* – 25–30% risk of malignant transformation

Spread

Local

- Chest wall
- Skin

Lymph

- Axilla
- Supraclavicular fossa, mediastinum

Blood

- Bone: Spine, Femur, Skull
- Liver
- Adrenal, ovaries, brain, peritoneum

Staging/prognosis

- Manchester study results
  - **Stage I** – lesion localized to breast
  - **Stage II** – stage I + mobile, ipsilateral axillary lymph nodes
  - **Stage III**
    - Skin involvement (*peau d'orange*)
    - Fixed to pectoral muscles
    - Fixed ipsilateral axillary nodes
    - Mobile/fixed ipsilateral supraclavicular nodes
  - **Stage IV**
    - Extensive skin involvement
    - Fixation to chest wall
    - Disease beyond affected breast/axilla/scf

TNM Classification

- **T1** – <2 cm
- **T2** – 2–5 cm
- **T3** – >5 cm
- **T4** – attached to skin/chest wall
- **N0** – no nodal metastases
- **N1** – ipsilateral mobile axillary nodes
- **N2** – ipsilateral fixed axillary nodes
- **N3** – supraclavicular nodes
- **M0** – no distant metastases
- **M1** – distant metastases

Prognostic indicators in breast cancer

- Stage (size of tumour, lymph node status, metastases)
- Grade
- Oestrogen receptor status
- Menopausal status

Survival most dependant on nodal involvement – 10YS

- No nodes – >75%
- 4+ nodes – <20%
- Stage I – 50%
- Stage II – 25%
- Stage III/IV – <5%

The grade of lesion also affects prognosis – high grade worsens prognosis.

Recurrent disease

- May occur 20–30 years after primary
- 8% of node-positive patients; 4% node-negative patients

Diagnosis

- History
- Examination
- Investigations
  - Mammography patients >50 years of age – atypical microcalcification or stromal pattern
  - Ultrasound (U/S) – patient <50 years of age
  - Fine Needle Aspiration (FNA)
  - Cytology (C5 = malignant; C4 = severe atypia; C3 = mild atypia; C2 = benign; C1 = not diagnostic)
  - Tru-cut or open biopsy (results still equivocal)

Treatment rationale

- Curative versus palliative aim

Curative

Local disease

- Wide local excision of tumour + radiotherapy or

or

- Mastectomy (may require small dose of adjuvant radiotherapy)

Nodal disease

- Obvious or known nodes – surgical axillary clearance (level III)
- No obvious nodes – axillary sample (level I or II)

Histology positive requires adjuvant radiotherapy

Axillary clearance
- Level I – axillary tail to lateral border of pectoralis major
- Level II – dissect to medial border of pectoralis minor
- Level III – apex of axilla (up to level of axillary vein)

- Risk of upper arm lymphoedema from excessive dissection, especially if radiotherapy administered
- Risk of residual disease in incomplete dissection

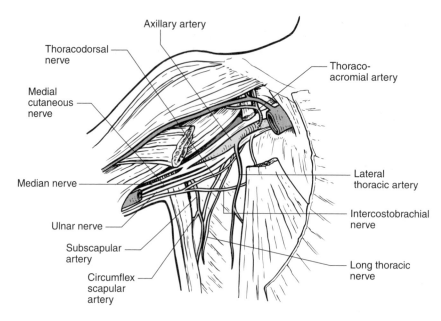

Figure 7.2 Anatomy of the axilla with pectoralis major and minor divided. From: *Fundamentals of Surgical Practice*; Greenwich Medical Media, 1998: page 352.

Systemic disease

- Premenopausal + nodes – adjuvant chemotherapy
- Post menopausal – tamoxifen for 5 years

Reconstructive and cosmetic

- Surgical improvement of cosmetic result
  - Implant
  - Latissimus dorsi or transrectus abdominus (TRAM) flap
- External support prosthesis

Palliative surgery

- Treat patient symptoms
  - Pain relief
  - Nausea, vomiting
- Control disease
  - Hormonal
    - Tamoxifen/Arimidex
    - Oophorectomy/adrenalectomy
  - Chemotherapy – 50–60% response

Note: Treatment policy depends on the individual patient and local policy.

Prevention

- High level media campaign on breast cancer awareness
- Screening programme

- Results to be evaluated
- Women 50–65 years of age invited for mammography
- Aim to detect non palpable or early lesions – will this improve survival figures?
- Problems with sensitivity and specificity of test
- Financial impact of programme
- Action on equivocal findings
  - Increased surgery for non-malignant disease?
  - Carcinoma *in situ*?

CARCINOMA *IN SITU*

- Natural history of lesion may vary in women

Ductal carcinoma *in situ* (DCIS)

- Preinvasive lesion? 30–50% risk of carcinoma in 10 years
- Treat with mastectomy +/– reconstruction
- High rate of recurrence in wide local excision of lesion (25–30%), 50% then become malignant

Lobular carcinoma *in situ* (LCIS)

- 25–30% of malignant change in 20 years
- 20% risk in 15 years
- 50% predisposed to ductal carcinoma
- Bilateral in 50–70% cases
- ?Mastectomy versus observation +/– tamoxifen

GYNAECOMASTIA

- Male breast enlargement – unilateral or bilateral
- Peak incidence in neonates puberty and >60 years of age

Causes

- Physiological
  - Neonatal – maternal oestrogens
  - Puberty – oestrogen/androgen imbalance
- Hypogonadism
  - Pituitary insufficiency
  - Androgen resistance
  - Kleinfelter's syndrome
  - Leprosy
- Neoplastic (*★produce ectopic hormones*)
  - Breast carcinoma
  - Testicular tumour★
  - Adrenal tumour★
  - Bronchial carcinoma★
- Hepatic – cirrhosis/liver failure
- Renal – dialysis

- Drugs
  - Cimetidine
  - Spironolactone
  - Stilboestrol
  - Cytotoxics
  - Isoniazid

BENIGN BREAST LUMPS

Developmental

- Fibroadenoma – common
  - Lobule hyperplasia single or multiple lesions
  - 15–40 years of age, 20% of benign breast disease exclude malignancy, if necessary excise
  - 1/1000 malignant change

Neoplastic

- Duct papilloma
  - Nipple discharge, often bloody, with associated lump
  - 35–40 years of age
  - Exclude malignancy, may require microdochectomy
- Neurofibroma
- Lipoma

Involutional

- >35 years of age, change in tissue, lobular to connective tissue transformation
- Fibrocystic disease
- Sclerosing adenosis
- Duct ectasia
- Simple hyperplasia

Inflammatory

- Abscess
  - Lactating/non-lactating
  - Treat with aspiration + antibiotics if possible
  - Incise and drain if not controllable
  - May form mammary fistula
- TB
- Syphillis
- Actinomycoses
- Herpes
- Periductal mastitis
- Fat necrosis – post-trauma

Hormonal

- Cyclical mastalgia, cyclical pain and nodularity of breasts

Note: in all cases exclude malignancy first.

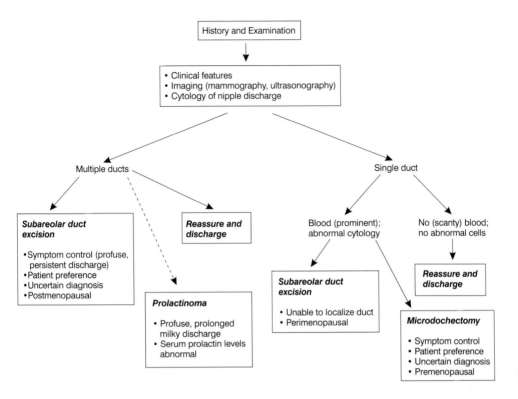

Figure 7.3 Management of a patient with nipple discharge.

THYROID

THYROID ENLARGEMENT (GOITRE)

- Malignant versus benign
- Assess Thyroid function – hyper/hypo/euthyroid

Indications for thyroidectomy

- Malignancy
- Obstruction
  - Airway compression (stridor/sleep apnoea)
  - Significant speech change
- Thyrotoxicosis – failure of medical management
- Retrosternal – risk of cystic bleeding, with large mediastinal vessel compression
- Cosmetic

THYROID SURGERY

- Total thyroidectomy – malignancy
- Subtotal thyroidectomy – thyrotoxicosis
- Partial throidectomy – benign localized lesion

Specific risks of surgery

Immediate

- Bleeding
  - Haematoma in confined space
  - Risk of airway compression
  - May need intubation and surgical re-exploration
- Laryngeal oedema – prolonged intubation required

Early

- Nerve palsy
  - Rec. laryngeal n.
  - Sup. laryngeal n. – voice changes
  - Sympathetic chain > (Horner's)
- Hypocalcaemia – removal of excess parathyroid tissue
- Thyrotoxic crisis
  - Manipulation of thyrotoxic gland (rare)
  - Distress, dyspnoea, tachcardia, hyperpyrexia, confusion
  - Treat – resuscitate, oxygen, anti-thyroid + β-blockers

Late

- Recurrent disease
- Hypothyroidism (in subtotal thyroidectomy for thyrotoxicosis)

INVESTIGATION OF THYROID DISEASE

History and examination

- Is the lesion a solitary nodule? Lesion within a multinodular colloid goitre
- Is the thyroid locally enlarged or diffusely enlarged?
- Is patient hyper/hypo/euthyroid?

Further assessment

- FNA – cytological evidence of lesion
- USS
  - Location of lesion
  - Presence of other lesions (eg MNCG)
- Isotope scan
  - Iodide–123 (half-life 13 h instead of I–131, 8 days)or technetium–99
  - Defines functionality of lesion
  - Most 'hot' nodules are benign
  - 80% of solitary lesions are cold, but only 10–20% are malignant
  - May locate ectopic thyroid tissue

Other

- CT/MRI
  - Retrosternal spread
  - Lymph nodes
- Tru-cut/open biopsy if diagnosis uncertain

Biochemistry

- T3, T4 and TSH
- Thyroid antibodies

CAUSES OF NON-MALIGNANT GOITRE

- Physiological
  - Pregnancy, lactation
  - Puberty
  - Endemic iodine deficiency
  - Dietary goitrogens contain thiocyanates, e.g. *Brassica* – cabbage, kale, rape
  - Dyshormonogenesis
- Drugs – propythiouracyl
- Autoimmune
  - Graves' disease (diffuse toxic goitre)
  - Hashimoto thyroiditis (hypothyroid)
- Other
  - De Quervains'(granulomatous thyroiditis)
  - Reidel's thyroiditis
  - Acute bacterial, chronic bacterial (TB, syphillis)
  - Amyloid

THYROID NEOPLASIA

Malignant thyroid neoplasia

- Overall incidence <4/100 000
- 0.5% all cancer deaths

Primary

Differentiated

- Papillary – 75% all thyroid tumours
  - Peak incidence 30–40 years, F>M 2:1
  - Higher incidence iodine rich areas, e.g. Iceland, neck irradiation
  - Spread via lymph nodes to cervical nodes (lateral aberrant thyroid); blood to lungs, bone
  - Total thyroidectomy +/– lymph node dissection +/– I–131 treatment
  - Good prognosis if intrathyroid (99% 5YS), extrathyroid >85% 5YS
- Follicular – 10% of thyroid tumours
  - Increase with age, >50 years, F>M
  - Low endemic iodine area, excess TSH stimulation, neck irradiation
  - Local invasion
  - Blood borne spread to bone, lungs: rare in lymph nodes
  - Total thyroidectomy +/– lymph node dissection +/– I–131 treatment
  - >95% 5YS if localized, 50% if invasive
- Medullary – 5–10%, F>M
  - From calcitonin-secreting parafollicular C-cells
  - Wide age range, familial (MEN II)
  - Lesion can secrete prostaglandins, serotonin, VIP, ACTH
  - Local invasion and lymph node spread
  - Total thyroidectomy +/– lymph node dissection +/– I–131 treatment
  - Monitor calcitonin levels
  - 50% 5YS if nodes positive

Undifferentiated anaplastic – <5%

- Elderly patients F>M
- May arise from pre-existing lesion or sporadic
- Rapid local invasion
- Rarely surgical option – palliative care only < 6 month mean survival

Malignant lymphoma – <5%

- Elderly, F>M
- Pre-existing thyroiditis (Hashimoto) or generalized lymphoma

Squamous cell carcinoma, sarcoma

- Rare
- 66% 5YS
- Secondary – local infiltration or blood borne spread

Benign thyroid neoplasia

- Follicular adenoma
  - Encapsulated solitary nodule or cyst
  - Lobectomy for confirmation of diagnosis
  - Small malignant potential
- Teratoma – rare

Thyroid cysts in MNCG (multinodular colloid goitre)

- Spontaneous enlargement causing
  - Rupture and possible infarction
  - Haemorrhage
  - Fibrosis
  - Calcification

Causes of thyrotoxicosis

- Diffuse toxic goitre (Graves' disease)
- Toxic multinodular goitre (Plummer's disease)
- Toxic adenoma
  - Overactive nodule
  - Autonomous activity, suppression of TSH > thyroid atrophy
- Rare – struma ovarii (thyroxine-secreting teratoma), metastatic thyroid cancer, pituitary adenoma secreting TSH

CONGENITAL THYROID ABNORMALITIES

- Lingual thyroid
  - Undescended thyroid tissue
  - Risk of hyperplasia and malignant change
- Thyroglossal cyst
  - Remnant of thyroglossal tract
  - Lined with stratified squamous epithelium + lymphoid tissue
  - Risk of malignant change
- Thyroglossal fistula – as for thyroglossal cyst

PARATHYROID DISEASE

- Normally 4 glands derived from IIIrd and IVth pharyngeal pouchs
- IIIrd pouch develops into thymus gland, migrating in mediastinum, non-consistent locations of parathyroids in neck
- Secrete parathormone (PTH)

ACTIONS OF PTH

- Stimulate osteoclastic activity leading to mobilization of calcium, phosphate
- Increased reabsorbtion of renal tubular calcium, increased excretion of phosphate
- Increased reabsorption of calcium from gut

HYPERPARATHYROIDISM

Primary

- Parathyroid adenoma (multiple in 6%) or hyperplasia
  - < 1% malignant transformation
  - local invasion
- High PTH and Ca^{2+} in serum
- Low PO_4, high alkaline phosphatase

Secondary

- Chronic renal failure or malabsorption
- Serum Ca low or normal

Tertiary

- Reactive hyperplasia and autonomy of parathyroids
- Glands no longer respond to physiological stimuli
- Original stimulus may have disappeared
- High serum Ca

Clinical features

Bone disease

- Decalcification
- Osteitis fibrosa cystica
  - Periosteal erosions
  - Pepperpot skull
  - Bone cysts

Kidney

- Stones

General

- Nausea, vomiting, anorexia
- Peptic ulcers, pancreatitis
- Tiredness, weakness
- Thirst, polyuria, weight loss

Investigations

- Serum Ca, PO_4, alkaline phosphatase
- Renal function
- PTH level
- Localization of lesion in primary hyperparathyroidism
  - CT/MRI scan
  - Thallium-technetium subtraction scan. Thallium taken up by thyroid and parathyroid, Technetium by thyroid only

Surgical treatment of parathyroid disease

The superior thyroid gland (IV) is normally found adjacent to the inferior thyroid artery and the inferior (III) adjacent to the lower pole of the thyroid gland. Of glands, 15% are ectopic (either adjacent to the superior thyroid vessels, the carotid sheath, within the thymus or the thyroid behind the larynx, pharynx or oesophagus or in the anterior or posterior mediastinum). In parathyroid hyperplasia three-and-a-half glands are removed and the remaining half is marked with a silk suture and autotransplanted into the muscles of the forearm, thus avoiding the need for neck re-exploration. Complications are the same as for thyroid surgery.

Other causes of hypercalcaemia
- Metastatic bone disease (breast, prostate, kidney, thyroid, bronchus)
- Multiple myeloma
- Ectopic PTH secretion (CA bronchus, kidney, ovary)
- Sarcoidosis
- Thyrotoxicosis
- Vitamin D intoxication

HYPOPARATHYROIDISM

- Post-thyroidectomy
- Removal or ischaemia of parathyroid tissue
- Symptoms when serum corrected Ca <2.00 mmol/l
  - Tingling of fingers, lips
  - Chvostek sign – tapping facial nerve angle of jaw leads to twitching of corner of mouth
  - Trousseau – cuff to forearm induces spasm
  - Treat with 10 ml 10% Ca gluconate infusion over 10 min

ADRENAL GLAND DISEASE

Adrenal glands situated bilaterally on upper poles of kidneys

Layer	Secretes
Outer adrenal cortex	
Zona glomerulosa	Mineralocorticoids, aldosterone
Zona fasciculata	Glucocorticoids, cortisol, corticosterone
Zona reticularis	Sex steroids, testosterone, oestrogen
Inner adrenal medulla	
Catecholamines	Adrenaline, noradrenaline

Investigations

- Serum electrolytes
- Serum aldosterone, cortisol levels
- Serum ACTH (distinguishes from pituitary dysfunction)
- Urinary steroid excretion
- Dexamethasone/metyrapone/synacthen tests
- CT/MRI scan

WORKUP OF AN INCIDENTAL ADRENAL MASS[4]

HYPERALDOSTERONISM

Primary (Conn's syndrome)

- Excess aldosterone secretion
- Na, H_2O retention causing hypertension, hypokalaemia
  - Aldosterone secreting adrenal adenoma
  - Bilateral adrenocortical hyperplasia
  - Ectopic aldosterone secreting tumour

Secondary – liver disease

HYPOADRENALISM

Acute

- Waterhouse–Friederichsen syndrome – bilateral adrenal haemorrhage in severe sepsis
- Post-bilateral adrenalectomy

Chronic

- Addison's disease
- Destruction of adrenal tissue – autoimmune, TB, metastatic CA, amyloid
- Muscular weakness, hypotension, irregular pigmentation of skin
- Treat medically

HYPERCORTICISM

ACTH dependant

- Pituitary adenoma (Cushing's) 80%
- Ectopic or iatrogenic ACTH

Non-ACTH dependant

- Adrenal neoplasm, adenoma/carcinoma
  - Carcinoma rare but highly malignant
  - Invasion of IVC, distal met
  - <20 5YS
- Hyperplasia
- Iatrogenic cortisol
- Clinical features – truncal obesity, thin skin, bruising, moon facies, buffalo hump, muscle wasting

DETERMINATION OF CAUSE OF CUSHING'S SYNDROME

Serum ACTH radioimmunoassay

- If ACTH is either not detectable or very low the patient has an autonomous adrenal tumour
- Serum ACTH is raised in Cushing's disease (pituitary-dependent bilateral adrenocortical hyperplasia) and it is very high in cases of ectopic ACTH production

Metapyrone test

- A large rise in plasma ACTH and urinary corticosteroids following metyrapone confirms a diagnosis of Cushing's disease

High dose dexamethasone suppression test

- A 50% suppression will occur in Cushing's disease but not in other causes of Cushing's syndrome

ADRENAL MEDULLA TUMOURS

- Chromaffin cells
  - Phaechromocytoma
    - 10%
      - Bilateral, malignant, extra-adrenal, multiple, familial in children
      - Extra-adrenal sites aortic bifurcation, renal hilum, chest neck
      - Higher incidence of malignancy (20–40%)
      - Part of MEN II syndrome
    - Paroxysmal or persistent hypertension
    - Palpitations, vomiting, sweating, dyspnoea, weakness, pallor
- Sympathetic neurones
  - Ganglioneuroma
    - Retroperitoneal sarcoma
    - Any age
  - Neuroblastoma

Preoperative preparation of a patient with phaeochromocytoma

- Adrenoceptor blockage
- Establish a-blockage that reduces vasoconstrictor tone and reduces systemic BP (using phenoxy benzamine or phentolamine) then use β-blockers to prevent tachycardia and arrythymias (propanolol)
- Restore blood circulation – reduced vasconstrictor tone produces an increased circulatory capacity (use i.v. fluids)

Intraoperative difficulties in a patient with a phaeochromocytoma

- Occlude the venous drainage of the tumour as excessive manipulation can cause a large catecholamine release leading to dramatic changes in blood pressure
- Intraoperative hypertensive crises are treated with nitroprusside
- Following removal of the tumour a profound fall in BP may occur, necessitating large volumes of intravenous fluid replacement

Treatment

Cushing's disease

- Bilateral adrenalectomy
- Pituitary irradiation should be given post operatively to prevent hyperpigmentation (Nelson's syndrome)
- Maintenance hydrocortisone and flurocortisone are required to prevent hypoadrenalism

Pituitary ablation for a hypophyseal tumour

- Hypophysectomy via a trans-sphenoidal or transfrontal route
- External beam pituitary radiation

Adrenal tumours

- Unilateral adrenalectomy for adenomas
- Bilateral adrenalectomy maybe required for synchronous adrenal carcinoma. Post operative radiotherapy is given to prevent recurrences and chemotherapy which inhibits the early stages of steroid biosynthesis is used to treat metastatic disease

Ectopic ACTH production

- The source of the ectopic secretion is removed after metyrapone preparation

MULTIPLE ENDOCRINE NEOPLASIA SYNDROMES

Inherited autosomal dominant disorder of APUD (amine precursor uptake and decarboxylation) cells.

MEN I
- Parathyroid hyperplasia (90%)
- Pancreatic Islet cell tumour (80%) – gastrin/insulin/glucagon/somstostatin/VIP secreting
- Pituitary adenoma (65%)

MEN IIA
- Parathyroid hyperplasia
- Medullary carcinoma of thyroid
- Phaeochromocytoma

MEN IIB – IIA and mucosal ganglioneuromas, marfanoid features, megacolon

8

TRANSPLANTATION

TRANSPLANT SURGERY

Historical landmarks in transplantation science

1902	Carrel	Renal transplantation in dogs, graft survival for 2 weeks Limited understanding of immune response
1936	Voronoy	Cadaver to human kidney transplant, patient survival 2 days
1942	Gibson and Medawar	Accelerated destruction of second skin grafts in burns patients Animal experiments demonstrating graft rejection phenomenon
1954	Murray (Boston)	First long-term successful transplantation identical twins (8 years of age) Twenty-nine further identical twin transplants, 20YS rate >50%
1961	Calne	Increased renal graft survival in dogs treated with 6- mercaptopurine Derivative azathioprine used in the Boston group
1963	Zukoski	Steroids improved graft survival in dog
1967	Starzl	First liver transplantation, Pittsburgh, longest survivor >20 years
1972	Borel	Immunosuppressive effect of 11 amino acid chain polypeptide cyclosporin A derived from *Cylindrocarpon lucidum* and *Tolypocladium inflatum* in a mouse model
1977	Calne	Cyclosporin effectiveness demonstrated in dog renal grafts

TISSUE TRANSPLANTATION AND 1 YEAR SURVIVAL (1YS) RATES

Kidney	Live	95%
	Cadaveric	75–90%
Liver		75%
Heart		75%
Heart–lung		70%
Lung		70%
Pancreas	Whole	60%
	Islet	poor
Cornea		95%
Skin/gut		Poor
Other tissues		
Blood		
Bone marrow		

IMMUNOLOGICAL CONSIDERATIONS

- Graft rejection
  - Hyper acute – hours, performed antibodies in sensitized recipient
  - Acute – days, cellular immune mechanism
  - Chronic – months/years, humoral mechanism
- Rejection rate reduced by
  - Tissue typing selection and matching
  - Pharmacological immunosuppression

TISSUE TYPING SELECTION AND MATCHING

- Determined by the major histocompatability complex (MHC)
- Located on human chromosome 6
- Class I antigens on most nucleated cells, encoded on HLA A, B and C regions of chromosome 6
- Class II antigens on activated T cells, antigen-presenting cells and B cells encoded on the HLA DR region of chromosome 6
- Matching of class I and II antigens allows cadaveric renal transplantation and a 1YS rate of 95% in the presence of chemical immunosuppression

GRAFT REJECTION

- Antigen presentation by antigen presenting cells (e.g. macrophage)
- Recognized by T-helper cells in the presence of the class II antigen on the surfaces of both cells
- Interaction then causes production of cytokines
- Macrophages release IL–1, then they act on T-helper cells to release cytokines IL–2 and interferons (IFN)
- Causes activation of other T cells (cytotoxic, inducer, suppressers) to effect immune response

PHARMOCOLOGICAL IMMUNOSUPPRESSION

- Triple therapy
  - Steroids (prednisolone) – inhibit IL–1 production
  - Azathioprine – interferes mRNA and DNA production
  - Cyclosporin – inhibits IL–2 release, spares suppresser T cells

Drug-induced side effects

- Steroids – Cushing's syndrome
- Cushing's facies, buffalo hump, central obesity, thin skin, bruising, proximal mypoathy, acne, hirsuitism
  - Avascular necrosis of hips
  - Cataracts
  - Diabetes
  - Hyperlipidaemia
  - Pancreatitis
  - Psychosis
- Azathioprine
  - Bone marrow suppression
  - Hepatotoxicity
- Cyclosporin
  - Nephrotoxicity
  - Hepatotoxicity
  - Tremors, convulsions
  - Hirsuitism, skin problems
  - Gingival hyperplasia
  - Hypertension

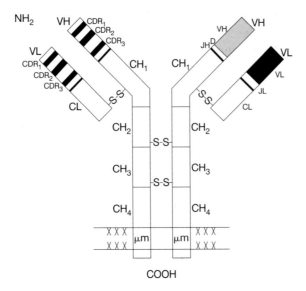

Figure 8.1 An immunoglobulin molecule. From: *Fundamentals of Surgical Practice*; Greenwich Medical Media, 1998: page 248.

- Malignant change >lymphoma
- Other drugs
  - OKT3 (anti-T cell monoclonal antibody)
  - FK 506

ORGAN DONATION CRITERIA

- Age
  - Kidney – 2–65 years
  - Liver – neonate–50 years
  - Heart – 15–45 years
- Absence of acute or chronic renal, hepatic, cardiac failure
- Absence of sepsis
- Hepatitis B and HIV-negative
- No malignancy (except primary brain lesion)
- Non diabetic
- CMV, HSV positive to positive recipients if possible

CRITERIA FOR DIAGNOSIS OF BRAIN DEATH[9]

- Precondition
  - Patient is in coma, receiving mechanical ventilation
  - Definitive diagnosis of the cause of coma
  - Enough time has elapsed to ensure irreversibility
  - Two doctors perform the tests independently (the doctors should be of senior rank and clearly identified)

- Exclusive criteria
  - The patient cannot be hypothermic (<35°C)
  - There must be no residual effects of sedative, anaesthetic, or neuromuscular relaxant drugs
  - Other metabolic or endocrine disease such as hypothyroidism, polyneuropathy, or myasthenia gravis must be excluded
- Signs
  - Unreactive pupils to bright light
  - Absent corneal reflexes
  - Absent vestibulo-ocular reflexes
  - No cold caloric responses (exclude ear wax)
  - 'Doll's eyes'
  - Absent purposeful movement
  - Absent motor response to pain stimulation
  - Absent decorticate or decerebrate posturing
  - Absent respiratory effect during formal apnoea test

Note: A formal document must be signed and dated, and the time of completion of testing recorded. If brain death is confirmed, this recorded time becomes the legal time of death.

CAUSES OF BRAIN DEATH LEADING TO ORGAN DONATION IN THE UK[8]

Condition	Percentage*
Intracranial haemorrhage/thrombosis/aneurysm	57.5
Trauma	
Road traffic accident	18
Other	7
Cardiac arrest including myocardial infarct	4
Brain tumour	2
Suicide	1.5
Asthma + other respiratory diseases	1
Other and unknown	9

*Data from the UK Transplant Support Service Authority

ORGAN STORAGE AND VIABILITY

Organ/tissue	Storage medium	Maximum storage time
Kidneys	ice	48–72 h
Liver	UW (University of Wisconsin) solution	20 h
Heart	ice	2–6 h
Lung	ice	1 h
Pancreas	UW	20 h
Cornea	4°C	48 h
Frozen + cryoprotectant		18 months

RECIPIENT

- Maximum age 70 years
- No existing cardiac/respiratory/renal/hepatic disease (other than system for transplantation)
- No malignancy
- No social or psychological contra-indication
- Patient willing to accept risks of surgery, complications including rejection and life time medication

KIDNEY TRANSPLANTATION

- More than 100,000 world-wide grafts

Indications

- Primary or secondary renal failure
  - Glomerulonephritis
  - Pyelonephritis
  - Polycystic disease
  - Diabetic kidney

  Note: May be in combination with pancreatic graft

Methods

- Living – related
- Cadaveric – full MHC match desirable
- General medical condition and renal function optimized with preoperative dialysis
- Extra peritoneal implantation into iliac fossae
- Ureter tunnelled into recipient bladder – ureteroneocystostomy
  - Drop-in/Politano–Leadbetter technique/myotomy/flush implantation
  - May require ileal conduit in neurogenic bladder or self catheterization

Surgical complications

Early
  - Anastomotic leak leading to haemorrhage
  - Renal vein/artery thrombosis
  - Ureteric leak

Late
  - Renal artery stenosis
  - Ureteric stenosis
  - Ureteric reflux

Causes of ureteric complications

- Damage to vascular supply
- Excessive damage/stripping of ureter
- Restrictive submucosal tunnel
- Rejection

Medical complications

- Rejection – hyperacute/acute/chronic
- Cyclosporin toxicity
- Acute tubular necrosis
- Systemic viral infection (CMV, HSV)
- Systemic or local bacterial sepsis (including pyelonephritis)
- Recurrence of primary disease

Postoperative and long-term care

- Monitor renal function
  - Urea, creatinine
  - Urine – protein, culture, cytology
  - Cyclosporin levels
  - General condition of patient
  - Graft U/S
  - Graft biopsy

Symptoms/signs of rejection

- General malaise
- Tenderness over graft
- Pyrexia

LIVER TRANSPLANTATION

- 10,000 in Europe
- 300–400 grafts/year in the UK

Indications

Acute liver failure

- Hepatitis A, B, Non A–non B
- Poisoning
  - Paracetamol
  - Anaesthetic agents
  - Rare drug reactions

Chronic liver failure

Cirrhosis

- Autoimmune
  - Chronic active hepatitis
  - Primary biliary cirrhosis
  - Sclerosing cholagitis
- Infective – hepatitis B
- Metabolic
- Wilson's disease
  - Haemachromatosis
- Other – alcohol

Primary liver tumours

Biliary atresia

Methods

- Storage in a UW solution of the donor graft
- Optimize recipient clotting immediately before operation
- Orthotopic implantation
  - Recipient liver removed
  - Veno–veno bypass
    - Decreased venous hypertension
    - Improved cardiac stability
    - Decreased blood loss
- Split liver grafting in a child recipient is possible
- Duct to duct with t-tube or Roux loop to small bowel can be used

Surgical complications

- Intraoperative haemorrhage
- Anastomotic leak
- Portal vein thrombosis
- Biliary leak
- Biliary stenosis

Medical complications and follow-up

As for renal.

PANCREATIC TRANSPLANTATION

Indications

- Severe insulin-dependent diabetes

Methods

- Islet cell – very poor results, research only
- Solid organ
  - Segmental or whole organ
  - Enteric or bladder drainage

Surgical complications

- Pancreatitis; fistula
- Venous thrombosis
- Anastomotic breakdown

SMALL BOWEL TRANSPLANTATION

Indications

- Patient on long-term total parenteral nutrition (TPN)*
- Short gut syndrome
  - Post-mesenteric infarction

- Resection following Crohn's disease
- Small bowel atresia/volvus

*See complications of TPN (page 24).

Specific problems

- Portal versus systemic drainage
- Graft versus host disease
- Patch rejection

Note: World experience shows high mortality and morbidity.

ETHICS IN TRANSPLANTATION

Organ shortage

- Perpetual shortage of donor organs
  - Kidney waiting list >5 years
  - Liver >6 months
- Patients may die or significantly deteriorate on waiting list
- Consent for organ donation
  - Who should be approached?
  - When should decision be made?
  - Criteria of brain death
- Commercialization of 'black market organs'
- Use of possible animal clones specifically for culture of organs

FINANCIAL ASPECTS

- Massive cost of transplantation programme
  - Multidisciplinary organization
  - Rapid matching/contact/surgical set-up required
  - Expensive and advanced level of medical and surgical backup
- Cost versus benefit argument
  - Renal dialysis – £15,000–20,000 per patient per year
  - Renal transplant – £10,000 one-off cost
  - Liver/heart transplantation – no medical alternative to surgery
  - Liver transplant – >£80,000–100,000 per patient
  - Home TPN – £25,000–30,000 per year

Note: No successful surgical rationale yet established.

9

UROLOGY

CONGENITAL ABNORMALITIES OF THE KIDNEY AND URETER[8]

- Renal aplasia
- Renal ectopia
  - Pelvic, kidney
  - Horseshoe kidney
  - Crossed dystopia
- Cystic disease
  - Polycystic kidneys
    - Infantile polycystic disease
    - Unilateral multicystic disease
  - Solitary cyst
- Aberrant renal vessels – multiple renal arteries and veins
- Duplication
  - Duplex kidneys
  - Duplex renal pelvis
  - Duplex kidney and ureter
- Others
  - Retrocaval ureter
  - Congenital megaureter
  - Ureterocoele

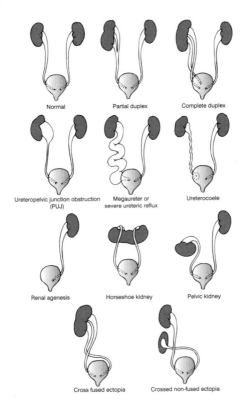

Figure 9.1 Common renal and ureteric congenital abnormalities.

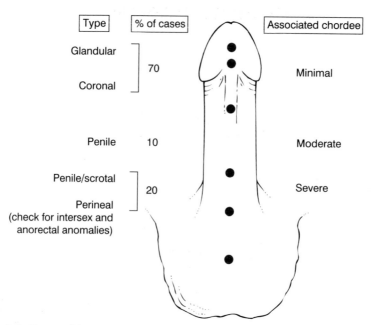

Figure 9.2 Types of hypospadius and associated degrees of chordee (a fibrous band that may cause bowing).

DIFFERENT TYPES OF KIDNEY INFECTIONS[8]

- Acute pyelonephritis
  - In childhood
  - In pregnancy
- With urinary obstruction
- Chronic pyelonephritis (reflux nephropathy)
- Pyonephrosis
- Renal abscess
- Perinephric abscess

INVESTIGATION OF UTI IN CHILDREN

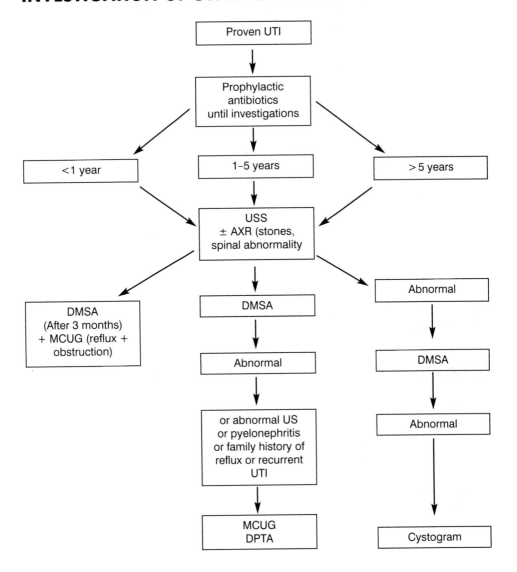

VESICOURETERIC REFLUX

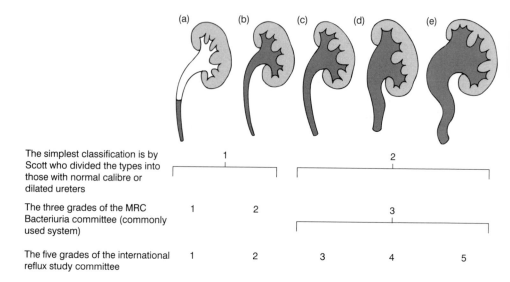

The simplest classification is by Scott who divided the types into those with normal calibre or dilated ureters — 1, 2

The three grades of the MRC Bacteriuria committee (commonly used system) — 1, 2, 3

The five grades of the international reflux study committee — 1, 2, 3, 4, 5

Figure 9.3 Grading of vesicoureteric reflux. Classification system has been inverted to include the simplest first International Reflux Study Committee grading (1–5). 1, Reflux into a non-dilated ureter; 2, reflux into the upper collecting system without dilatation; 3, reflux into a dilated ureter and/or blunting of the calyces; 4, reflux into a grossly dilated ureter; 5, massive reflux with ureteral dilatation, tortuosity and effacement of the calyceal details.

Note: When the ureter is dilated and/or associated with a para-ureteric diverticulum then reflux is unlikely to cease spontaneously and reimplantation should be considered. Grading Vesicoureteric Reflux; Grade I Ureters only, no dilatation; Grade II Up to the pelvis; Grade III + dilatation; Grade IV into the kidneys; Grade V)

Indications for surgery in vesico-ureteric reflux[2]

- Poor response to antibiotics or breakthrough infections
- Poor follow up or compliance to antibiotic treatment
- Associated abnormalities: excessive ballooning of pelvis on voiding, ureter duplication, para-ureteral saccules and gaping ureteric orifices
- Persistence of reflux into puberty

HAEMATURIA

- Microscopic haematuria is the presence in urine of >5–10 red blood cells at 200× magnification and must be distinguished from haemoglobinuria and myoglobinuria
- A definite aetiology will be established in 60–70% of patients presenting with haematuria

CAUSES OF HAEMATURIA BY PATHOLOGY[2]

- Tumours – renal parenchyma, urothelium, prostate (35%)
- Infections – bacterial, TB, parasitic (30%)
- Trauma (9%)
- Calculi – renal, ureteric or bladder (9%)
- Congenital – hydronephrosis, renal cysts, polycystic disease (5%)
- Stricture (5%)
- Bleeding diatheses – haemophilia, thrombocytopenia, sickle cell disease (4%)
- Drugs – anticoagulants, cyclophosphamide, penicillamine (4%)
- Miscellaneous – exercise, prostatic varices (4%)
- 'Medical' – glomerulonephritis, renal emboli, renal vein thrombosis

CAUSES OF HAEMATURIA BY SITE[12]

Kidney
- Glomerular disease
- Polycystic kidneys
- Carcinoma
- Stone
- Trauma including renal biopsy
- Tuberculosis
- Embolism (from myocardial infarct, SBE)
- Renal vein thrombosis
- Vascular malformation

Ureter
- Stone
- Neoplasm

Bladder
- Carcinoma
- Stone
- Trauma
- Inflammatory – cystitis, TB
- Bilharzia

Prostate
- BPH
- Neoplasm

Urethra
- Trauma
- Stone
- Urethritis
- Neoplasm

General
- Anticoagulants
- Thrombocytopenia
- Haemophilia
- Sickle cell disease
- Malaria
- Purpura
- Scurvy

RENAL CALCULI

- General practice incidence of stones in males of 45–60 years of age is 21/10,000[1]

RELATIVE INCIDENCE OF STONE TYPES[2]

- Pure calcium oxalate – (45%) hard irregular and brittle
- Calcium oxalate + phosphate – (25%) hard irregular and brittle
- Triple phosphate (calcium, magnesium and phosphate) – (20%) infective white, soft and staghorns

- Uric acid – (5%) radiolucent* yellow
- Calcium phosphate (3%)
- Cystine, pure oxalate (3%)

*10% of renal calculi are radioluscent.

IDENTIFIABLE CAUSES OF RENAL CALCULUS FORMATION[2]

- Idiopathic hypercalciuria – 65%
- Urinary infection – 20%
- Cystinuria – 5%
- Hyperparathyroidism – 4%
- Medullary sponge kidney – 3%
- Hyperoxaluria – 2%
- Hyperuricosuria – 2%
- Urinary diversion – <1% (including ileostomy)
- Other/unknown – 5–10%
  - Steroids
  - Sarcoidosis
  - Milk alkali syndrome
  - Hypervitaminosis D
  - Renal tubular acidosis
  - Prolonged immobilization
  - Multiple myelomatosis

Note: the majority of patients harbouring calculi have no detectable anatomical, biochemical or metabolic abnormality.

Usual sites of stone hold up

- Pelviureteric junction
- Pelvic brim
- Vesicoureteric junction

Probability of a stones passing related to size[4]

- 60% of renal stones pass spontaneously (half within the first 24 h)
- 90% of 4 mm stones in the distal ureter pass
- 90% of 5 mm stones within 5 cm of the vesco ureteric junction pass spontaneously; 50% of 7 mm stones in the proximal or distal ureter pass
- A stone will rarely pass if >7 mm size in the mid-ureter and only 20% of 8 mm stones in the distal ureter will pass

---

PATHOLOGICAL EFFECTS OF RENAL AND URETERIC CALCULI[2]

- Recurrent infections with pyelonephritis
- Cortical scarring and atrophy
- Haematuria

- Hydroureter
- Oedema and periureteric inflammation
- Hydronephrosis
- Perinephric abscess
- Hydrocalcinosis
- Extravasation of urine

MEDICAL TREATMENT OF STONE DISEASE[2]

- Unless the underlying metabolic defect is corrected after removal of the stone 70% of patients will develop a recurrence within 10 years
- General – avoid dehydration, increase overall fluid intake and reduce consumption of protein rich foods and calcium containing foods
- Specific
  - Calcium oxalate – hypercalciuria (excessive dietary intake of calcium, absorptive due to increased protein or phosphates, resorptive from immobilization or primary hyperparathyroidism (2% of stone formers), tubular from secondary hyperparathyroidism, idiopathic by far form the largest group
    Treatment – thiazide diurectics impair calcium secretion and oral cellulose phosphate prevent absorption
  - Triple phosphate – *Proteus* splits urea into ammonia which alkalinizes the urine encouraging precipitation of calcium salts
    Pyrophosphate an inhibitor of crystallization is found in decreased concentration
    Treatment – antibiotics and acidification of the urine
  - Uric acid – stones occur in 25% of patients with gout. Their urinary pH is low, uric acid secretion is raised and deficient in acidic mucopolysaccharide (a specific inhibitor of crystallization)
    Treatment – reducing purine dietary intake, alkalizing the urine with 3–6 g per day of sodium bicarbonate and the addition of allopurinol at 200–400 mg per day
  - Cysteine – stones form in patients who have autosomal recessive abnormalities in reabsorption of cysteine, ornithine, arginine and lysine (COAL). Cysteine crystals in urine are pathological
    Treatment – urinary alkalization with sodium bicarbonate and oral penicillamine can cause dissolution
  - Oxalate (pure) – hyperoxaluria can be secondary to malabsorptive syndromes, e.g. short bowel but most stones are due a genetic failure of glycosylase or hydroxypyruvate
    Treatment – alkaline citrate, reduce fat intake, calcium if low calcium excretion, pyridoxine if B_6 deficient

COMMON SURGICAL TREATMENT OF STONE DISEASE[4]

- Extracorporeal shock wave lithotrypsy (ESWL) – shock waves are focused by an ellipsoid reflector on to the stone.
- Percutaneous nephrosto lithotomy (PCNL) – graded dilators are passed over a fine wire placed in the kidney until a nephroscope can be passed into the renal pelvis. The stone can then be removed intact, be crushed or disintegrated by ultrasound or an electrohydraulic probe.
- Ureteroscopy – direct visualization via a fine fibreoptic scope allows baskets to entrap lower third stones, and middle or upper third stones can be pushed back into the kidney for PCNL (push–pull) or ESW (push–bang).
- Open surgery or a mixture of modalities.

CRITERIA IN DECISION-MAKING OF TYPE OF TREATMENT FOR URINARY CALCULI[4]

- Stone factors
  - Single stone 25–30 mm – Rx: PCNL
  - Multiple total size 25–30 mm – Rx: ESWL
- Anatomic urinary factors
  - Inaccessible ureteric orifices
  - Lower pole calculi are less amenable to ESWL and more amenable to PCNL
- Extra urinary factors – pregnancy, bleeding diathesis, obesity (i.e. patient factors)

Therefore:

- Ureteroscopy is commonly used in lower ureteral stones
- ESWL is commonly used in renal and upper ureteral calculi (and it can treat 90% of all stones)
- PCNL is commonly used in staghorn or large single calculi of 2.5 cm and for cysteine calculi which are often resistant to ESWL

INDICATIONS FOR SURGICAL REMOVAL OF A URETERIC CALCULUS[8]

- Repeated attacks of pain and the stone is not moving
- Stone is enlarging
- Complete obstruction of the kidney
- Urine is infected
- Stone is too large to pass
- Stone is obstructing a solitary kidney or there is bilateral obstruction

KIDNEY

COMMON CAUSES OF AN ENLARGED KIDNEY[12]

- Hydronephrosis
- Pyonephrosis
- Perinephric abscess
- Malignant disease – carcinoma of the kidney and nephroblastoma
- Solitary cysts
- Polycystic disease
- Hypertrophy

Causes of a renal masses

Benign	Malignant
• Simple cysts	• Renal cell carcinoma
• Multiple cysts	• Transitional cell carcinoma
• Tubular ectasia	• Squamous cell carcinoma
• Dermoid	• Nephroblastoma
• Lipoma, angioma, leiomyoma	• Sarcoma
• TB	• Metastatic (lung, breast)
• Angiomyolipomata (50% are associated with tuberous sclerosis)	

TYPES OF RENAL TUMOUR[2,1]

Renal parenchyma

- Benign (rare)
  - Adenoma
  - Fibroma
  - Haemangioma
  - Angiomyolipoma
  - Mesoblastic nephroma
- Malignant
  - Renal adenocarcinoma (hypernephroma, Grawitz) 80% of all renal tumours
  - Nephroblastoma (Wilms' tumour see paediatric tumours)
  - Sarcoma
  - Metastases (lung breast or stomach)
  - Lymphoma
  - Melanoma

Renal pelvis

- Benign (rare) – papilloma
- Malignant
  - Transitional cell carcinoma
  - Squamous cell carcinoma
  - Adenocarcinoma

RENAL CELL CARCINOMA (HYPERNEPHROMA)

- Males are affected twice as commonly as females. Increased incidence in smokers, coffee drinkers, industrial exposure to exposure cadmium, lead, asbestos, aromatic hydrocarbon, renal cysts in dialysis patients, von Hippel–Lindau disease.
- Spread is by direct extension into perinephric tissues, by lymphatics to the para-aortic nodes, along the renal vein to bone, liver and brain, and cannon ball metastases in the lung.
- History.

ASSOCIATED SYNDROMES OF RENAL CELL TUMOURS[2]

- Raised ESR – 53%
- Weight loss and fatigue – 48%
- Anaemia – 43%
- Abnormal LFT – 15%
- Fever (PUO) – 15%
- Hypertension – 15%
- Erythrocytosis – 4% (excess erythrpoietin)
- Hypercalcaemia – 4% (ectopic parathyroid hormone)
- Neuromyopathy – 3%
- Amyloidosis – 3%
- Hepatomegaly, breathlessness and pathological fractures due to secondaries
- Investigations – urine analysis for blood, Hb, FBC-anaemia, polycythaemia due to erythropoietin production, ESR – raised, Us, CXR to exclude metastases, IVU – distorted calyces and calcification, CT scan, angiogram – tumour circulation versus cyst

STAGING OF RENAL TUMOURS

Stage	Description	5-Year survival (%)	10-Year survival (%)	Treatment
I	Confined within the capsule	65	56	Resectable
II	Into perirenal fat (Gerota fascia intact)	47	20	Resectable
III	Into renal vein (+/– perinephric/lymph node involvement)	51	37	Unresectable*
IV(A)	Adjacent organ involvement (excluding adrenal)	8 overall	7 overall	Unresectable*
IV(B)	Distant metastases			

*IL2 can be given as adjuvant therapy in non-localized disease, radiotherapy can palliate metastatic pain. Follow up is indefinite.

CAUSES OF UNILATERAL URETERIC OBSTRUCTION[8]

Extramural obstruction

- Tumour from adjacent structures, e.g. carcinoma of the cervix, prostate, rectum, colon or caecum
- Idiopathic retroperitoneal fibrosis
- Retrocaval ureter

Intramural obstruction

- Congenital stenosis, physiological narrowing of the pelvi-ureteric junction, leading to pelviureteric junction obstruction
- Ureterocele and congenital small ureteric orifice
- Inflammatory stricture following removal of a calculus, repair of a damaged ureteric segment or tuberculous infection
- Neoplasm of the ureter or bladder cancer involving the ureteric orifice

Intraluminal obstruction

- Calculus in the renal pelvis or ureter
- Sloughed papilla in papillary necrosis (especially in diabetic individuals, analgesic abusers and those with sickle-cell disease, may obstruct the ureter)

BLADDER

BLADDER CALCULI

Aetiology
- Children (India, Thailand, Egypt, Turkey) – severe dehydration causes formation of uric acid stones
- Adult
  - Outflow obstruction

- Chronic infection
- Foreign body
- Upper tract stone
- Investigation – KUB and cystoscopy
- Treatment
  - Underlying abnormality
  - Electrohydraulic lithotrypsy or crushing lithoclast for smaller stoned
  - Open lithotomy for stones >5 cm
  - Cystoscopy post-stone removal to exclude squamous carcinoma of the bladder

BLADDER CANCER

Factors implicated in development of urothelial cancers[2]

- Occupational exposure (2-naphthlamine, 4-aminodiphenyl, benzidine, magenta and auramine dyes)
- Cigarette smoking (doubles the risk)
- Drugs phenacetin/aspirin, cyclophosphamide
- Associated disease – schistosomiasis, Balkan nephropathy ($\times$ 200 risk), exstrophy (ectopia vesicae), leukoplakia, urachal remnants, pelvic irradiation
- Endogenous carcinogens nitrosamines, tryptophane metabolites
- Chronic inflammation bladder outflow obstruction + infection + stones/diverticulum

---

Occupations that have exposed workers at some time to urothelial carcinogens[6]

- Chemical dye manufacture
- Rubber industry
- Leather industry
- Electric cable manufacture
- Gas production in vertical retort houses
- Rodent operators (rat catchers)
- Patent fuel manufacture
- Laboratory work
- Sewage and water testing

Types of urothelial tumour[2]

Malignant

- Transitional cell carcinoma (90%) occurs in the bladder, 97%, renal pelvis, 2% and ureters, 1%
- Squamous cell carcinoma (5–8%)
- Adenocarcinoma (1–2%)
- Undifferentiated carcinoma
- Sarcoma

Benign

- Papilloma (0.5%)
- Fibro epithelial polyp
- Symptoms and signs – painless haematuria, dysuria, frequency and urgency. Hydronephrosis, CRF. Pain from pelvic invasion

- Investigations – Hb, FBC, ESR, U&Es, creatinine, MSU, urine cytology, BTaStat, IVU-filling defects, hydronephrosis, USS, EUA to assess tumour spread, (flexible) cystoscopy and biopsy, CXR, CT scan to determine spread, bone scan to determine metastases

Treatment of bladder tumours

TNM clinical classification for tumours of the bladder7

- **T** – primary tumour
- **Tx** – primary tumour cannot be assessed
- **T0** – no evidence of primary tumour
- **Ta** – non-invasive papillary carcinoma
- **Tis** – carcinoma *in situ*: 'flat tumour'
- **T1** – tumour invades subepithelial connective tissue
- **T2a** – tumour invades superficial muscle (inner half)
- **T2b** – tumour invades deep muscle (outer half)
- **T3a** – tumour invades perivesical tissue (microscopically)
- **T3b** – tumour invades perivesical tissue (macroscopically)
- **T4** – tumour invades any of the following: prostate, uterus, vagina, pelvic wall, abdominal wall
- **T4a** – tumour invades prostate, uterus, vagina
- **T4b** – tumour invades pelvic wall, abdominal wall
- **N** – regional lymph nodes
- **Nx** – regional lymph nodes cannot be assessed
- **N0** – no regional lymph nodes metastasis
- **N1** – metastasis in a single lymph node ≤ 2 cm in greatest dimension
- **N2** – metastasis in a single lymph node >2 cm and <5 cm in greatest dimension, or multiple lymph nodes, none >5 cm in greatest dimension
- **N3** – metastasis in a lymph node >5 cm in greater dimension
- **M** – distant metastasis
- **Mx** – presence of distant metastasis cannot be assessed
- **M0** – no distant metastasis
- **M1** – distant metastasis

*The suffix (m) should be added to the appropriate T category to indicate multiple tumours. The suffix (is) may be added to any T to indicate the presence of associated carcinomas *in situ*.

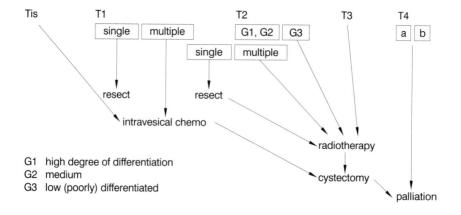

G1 high degree of differentiation
G2 medium
G3 low (poorly) differentiated

Prognosis of bladder tumours

Stage	5-Year survival
Ta	90–100%
T1	70%
T2	55%
T3	35%
T4	10–20%

5-YS is related to grade:
- I – well differentiated no invasion: 90%
- II – 30%

METHODS OF URINARY DIVERSION

These can classified as:
- Temporary or permanent
- Intubated or non-intubated
- Vesical or non-vesical

and include:
- Nephrostomy
- Ureterostomy *in situ*
- Loop cutaneous ureterostomy
- End cutaneous ureterostomy
- Trans uretero-ureterostomy
- Suprapubic cystostomy
- Cutaneous vesicostomy
- Isolated ileal conduit
- Continent urinary reservoir
- Uretro-sigmoidostomy
- Isolated colon circuit
- Rectal bladder

FUNCTIONAL CLASSIFICATION OF VOIDING DYSFUNCTION[4]

Failure to store

Because of bladder
- Detrusor hyperactivity
  - Involuntary contraction
    - Suprasacral neurological disease
    - Bladder outlet obstruction
    - Idiopathic
  - Decreased compliance
    - Fibrosis
    - Idiopathic

- Sensory urgency
  - Inflammatory
  - Infectious
  - Neurological
  - Psychological
  - Idiopathic

Because of outlet

- Stress incontinence
- Non-functional bladder neck/proximal urethra (intrinsic sphincter dysfunction)

Failure to empty

Because of bladder

- Neurological
- Myogenic
- Psychogenic
- Idiopathic

Because of outlet

- Anatomical
  - Prostatic obstruction
  - Bladder neck contracture
  - Urethral stricture
- Functional
  - Smooth sphincter dyssynergia
  - Striated muscle dyssynergia

CLASSIFICATION OF INCONTINENCE[4]

- Urethral
  - Due to lack of awareness of concern
  - Bladder abnormalities
    - Hyperactivity
      - Involuntary contractions
      - Decreased compliance
      - Sensory urgency and incontinence
  - Outlet abnormalities
    - Urethral instability
    - Stress incontinence
    - Non-functioning bladder neck/proximal urethra
  - Overflow incontinence
- Extra urethral
  - Fistula
  - Ectopic urethra

THERAPY TO FACILITATE URINE STORAGE[4]

Inhibiting bladder contractility/decreasing sensory input/increased bladder capacity

- Timed bladder emptying

- Pharmacologic therapy
  - Anticholinergic agents
  - Musculotropic relaxants
  - Calcium antagonists
  - Potassium channel openers
  - Prostaglandin inhibitors
  - β-Adrenergic agonists
  - Tricyclic antidepressants
  - Dimethyl sulphoxide
- Biofeedback, bladder retraining
- Bladder over distention
- Electrical stimulation
- Interruption of innervation
  - Central (subarachnoid block)
  - Peripheral (sacral rhizotomy, selective sacral rhizotomy)
  - Dorsal rhizotomy; dorsal root ganglionectomy
  - Perivesical (peripheral bladder denervation)
- Augmentation cystoplasty

Increasing outlet resistance

- Physiotherapy, biofeedback
- Pharmacologic therapy
  - α-Adrenergic agonists
  - Tricyclic antidepressants
  - β-Adrenergic agonists
  - Oestrogen
- Vesicourethral suspension
- Bladder outlet reconstruction
- Surgical mechanical compression
  - Sling procedures
  - Artificial urinary sphincter
- Non-surgical mechanical compression
  - Periurethral polytef injection
  - Periurethral collagen injection
  - Occlusive devices
- Electrical stimulation of the pelvic floor

Circumventing the problem

- Antidiuretic hormone-like agents
- Intermittent catheterization
- Continuous catheterization
- Urinary diversion
- External collecting devices
- Absorbent products

THERAPIES TO FACILITATE BLADDER EMPTYING[4]

Increasing intravesical pressure/bladder contractility

- External compression. Valsalva manoeuvre
- Promotion or initiation of reflex contractions

- Trigger zones or manoeuvres
- Bladder training, tidal drainage
- Pharmacologic therapy
  - Parasympathomimetic agents
  - Prostaglandins
  - Blockers of inhibition
    - α-Adrenergic antagonists
    - Opoid antagonists
- Reduction cystoplasty
- Electrical stimulation
  - Directly to the bladder or spinal cord
  - To the nerve roots
  - Transurethral intravesical electrotherapy

Decreasing outlet resistance

- At site of anatomic obstruction
  - Prostatectomy
  - Balloon dilatation
  - Intraurethral stent
  - Decrease prostatic size of tone
    - Luteinizing hormone releasing hormone agonists
    - Anti-androgens
    - α-Reductase inhibitor
    - α-Adrenergic antagonists
  - Urethral stricture repair/dilatation
- At the level of the smooth sphincter
  - Transurethral resection or incision of the bladder neck
  - Y–V plasty of the bladder neck
  - Pharmacological therapy
    - α-Adrenergic antagonists
    - β-Adrenergic agonists
- At the level of the striated sphincter
  - Surgical sphincterotomy, botulinum A toxin
  - Urethral over dilatation
  - Urethral stent
  - Pudendal nerve interruption
  - Pharmological therapy
    - Skeletal muscle relaxants
      - Benzodiazepines
      - Baclofen
      - Danrolene
    - α-Adrenergic antagonists
  - Psychotherapy, biofeedback

Circumventing the problem

- Intermittent catheterization
- Continuous catheterization
- Urinary diversion

URINARY TRACT OBSTRUCTION

CAUSES OF URINARY TRACT OBSTRUCTION IN GENERAL[1,5]

From outside

- Pelviureteric compression (bands, aberrant vessels)
- Tumours, e.g. retroperitoneal growth, glands, carcinoma of colon, diverticulitis, aortic aneurysm)
- Retroperitoneal fibrosis (primary, secondary to AAA or tumour)
- Iatrogenic, accidental ligation of the ureter at hysterectomy, colectomy
- Retrocaval ureter (right sided obstruction)
- Prostatic obstruction
- Bladder diverticulum
- Pregnancy
- Inflammation secondary to diverticulitis, Crohn's, appendicitis
- Congenial cysts (lower pole kidney, mesenteric, urachal)
- Pelvic tumours, e.g. carcinoma of the cervix
- Phimosis

Within the wall

- Pelvi-ureteric muscular dysfunction/PUJ obstruction (congenital 10% bilateral)
- Ureteral stricture (TB especially post-treatment, calculus, schistosomiasis)
- Congenital mega ureter
- Congenital bladder neck obstruction
- Neuropathic bladder
- Urethral stricture (calculus, gonococcal, post-instrumentation)
- Tumour, sarcoma
- Congenital urethral valve
- Pin hole meatus

Within lumen

- Calculus
- Blood clot
- Sloughed papilla (diabetes, analgesic abuse, sickle cell disease)
- Tumours of renal pelvis or ureter
- Bladder tumour

CAUSES OF BLADDER OUTFLOW OBSTRUCTION[2,4]

Congenital

- Urethral valves (anterior and posterior)
- Urethral polyps
- Urethral stricture

Acquired

- Structural
  - Benign prostatic disease
  - Carcinoma of the prostate
  - Bladder neck stenosis
  - Urethral stricture

- Urethral carcinoma
- Urethral calculi/mucus
- External compression (faecal impaction, pelvic tumour, distended uterus)
- Functional
  - Bladder neck dyssynergia
  - Detrusor-sphincter dyssynergia
  - Neurological disease (spinal cord injuries, spinal cord disease, e.g. tabes dorsalis, spinal tumour, MS, diabetic autonomic neuropathy)
  - Drug (anticholinergics, antidepressants) or alcohol toxicity
  - Pain (nociceptor retention, i.e. postoperative, post-trauma)

PROSTATE AND URETHRA

BENIGN PROSTATIC HYPERTROPHY

Symptoms of 'prostatism'[8]

'Obstructive'	'Irritative'
• Hesitancy (worsened if the bladder is very full) • Poor flow (unimproved by straining) • Intermittent stream – stops and starts • Dribbling (including after micturition) • Sensation of poor bladder emptying • Episodes of near retention	Frequency Nocturia Urgency Urge incontinence Nocturnal incontinence (enuresis)

- Other symptoms of BPH include:
- Haematuria from dilated bladder neck veins, palpable bladder, enlarged kidneys due to hydronephrosis, signs of uraemia and a smooth enlarged prostate on PR
- Investigations – Hb, FBC, U&E, creatinine, PAP and PSA to exclude malignancy, MSU, USS to assess if hydronephrosis of the upper tracts exists and measure post-voiding residual urine

Treatment options for BPH[4]

- Observation (watchful waiting)
- Pharmacologic
  - Bulk reducing
    - Luteinizing hormone releasing hormone agonist
    - Anti-androgen
    - 5a-reductase inhibitor
  - Tone reducing – α–1-adrenergic antagonists
- Surgical/mechanical
  - Urethral stent
  - Balloon dilatation
  - Transurethral or interstitial thermotherapy
  - Laser prostatotomy/prostatectomy
  - Interstitial laser application

- Diathermy prostatotomy (transurethral incision of the bladder neck-prostate [BNI])
- TURP
- Open prostatectomy

PROSTATIC CARCINOMA

This is the third most common malignancy in males. Spread occurs to adjacent organs, e.g. bladder, urethra and seminal vesicles. Lymphatic spread occurs to the iliac and para-aortic nodes and early via the blood, especially to the pelvis, spine and skull producing osteosclerotic lesions.

Symptoms and signs

The majority are asymptomatic, but obstructive symptoms and metastatic symptoms can occur. These include anaemia, weight loss, bone pain, pathological fractures, sciatica and weight loss. Rectal examination may reveal a hard (indurated) mass with in the prostate, bone pain and hepatomegaly.

Investigations

- Similar to BPH but including plain films for metastases in lungs and ribs, pelvis, spine or skull, bone scan, transrectal ultrasound and biopsy[15]

TNM classification of prostate cancer[7]

- **T** – primary tumour
- **Tx** – primary tumour cannot be assessed
- **T0** – no evidence of primary tumour
- **T1** – clinically unapparent tumour, not palpable or visible by imaging
- **T1a** – tumour an incidental histological finding in 5% or less of tissue resected
- **T1b** – tumour an incidental histological finding in > 5% of tissue resected
- **T1c** – tumour identified by needle biopsy (e.g. because of elevated prostate-specific antigen, PSA)
- **T2** – tumour confined within prostate
- **T2a** – tumour involves half a lobe or less
- **T2b** – tumour involves more than half a lobe but not both lobes
- **T2c** – tumour involves both lobes
- **T3** – tumour extends through the prostatic capsule
- **T3a** – extracapsular extension, unilateral or bilateral
- **T3b** – tumour invades seminal vesicle(s)
- **T4** – tumour is fixed or invades adjacent structures other than seminal vesicles
- **N** – regional lymph nodes
- **Nx** – regional lymph nodes cannot be assessed
- **N0** – no regional lymph node metastasis
- **N1** – metastasis in a single lymph node $\leq$ 2 cm in greatest dimension
- **N2** – metastasis in a single lymph node, >2 cm $\leq$ 5 cm in greatest dimension, or multiple lymph nodes, none >5 cm in greatest dimension

- **N3** – metastasis in a lymph node >5 cm in greatest dimension
- **M** – distant metastasis
- **Mx** – presence of distant metastasis cannot be assessed
- **M0** – no distant metastasis
- **M1** – distant metastasis
- **M1a** – non-regional lymph node(s)
- **M1b** – bone(s)
- **M1c** – other site(s)

- Tumour found in one or both lobes by needle biopsy, but not palpable or visible by imaging is classified as T1c
- Invasion into the prostatic apex or into (but not beyond) the prostatic capsule is not classified as T3 but as T2
- When more than one site of metastasis is present, the most advanced should be used for staging

Treatment of prostatic carcinoma

- Localized disease – surveillance and androgen ablation is at present the most common treatment in the UK for older patients (> 70 yrs). Radical treatment (either 'nerve sparing' prostatectomy or radiotherapy) is controversial and usually reserved for the younger patients
- Advanced tumours
  - Androgen ablation
  - Bilateral subcapsular orchiectomy
  - Diethylstlbesterol
  - DHT/testosterone receptor blockage
  - LHRH agonists
  - Aminoglutethimide and ketoconazole (second line medication)

Prognosis of prostatic tumours

- Patients with small primary localized lesions (T0–T1, N0, M0) have 70–75% 10YS
- Larger primary lesions T2–T3 are associated with a 50% 5YS
- Patients with metastatic, M1 have a 25% 5YS and a 10% 10YS

Urethral stricture[2]

Aetiology

- Congenital

Common congenital abnormalities of the male urethra[8]
- Meatal stenosis
- Congenital urethral stricture
- Congenital valves
- Hypospadias
- Epispadias

- Acquired
  - Traumatic
    - Instrumentation (indwelling catheter, endoscopy)
    - Rupture/trauma (iatroenic, open prostatectomy, amputation of the penis)

- Infective
  - Gonococcal
  - Non-specific urethritis
  - Syphilis (post-urethral chance)
  - TB
- Inflammatory
  - Balanitis xerotica obliterans (meatal) BXO
  - Chemical urethritis (catheter)
- Neoplastic
  - Squamous cell carcinoma
  - Transitional cell carcinoma
  - Adenocarcinoma

Treatment of urethral stricture[5]

- Dilatation
  - Gum-elastic bougie
  - Filiform and follower
  - Metal sounds
  - Self dilation with Nelaton catheter
- Urethrotomy
  - Internal visual urethrotomy
  - External urethrotomy
- Urethroplasty
  - Excision of the stricture and end-to-end anastomosis
  - Patch urethroplasty

PENIS

INDICATIONS FOR CIRCUMCISION[10]

- Religious
- Phimosis
- Paraphimosis
- Recurrent balanoprosthitis
- Diagnosis of underlying penile tumours
- Trauma and tumour of the foreskin

SQUAMOUS CELL CARCINOMA OF THE PENIS[4]

This is rare and almost unknown in the circumcised male. Poor hygiene and accumulation of smegma may be aetiological factors. Erythroplasia of Queyrat (a red velvety lesion of the glans) is premalignant. Tumour starts in the sulcus between the glans and foreskin and spreads to the inguinal nodes.

Signs and symptoms

- Firm, ulcerated, painless lesions, offensive blood stained discharge, inguinal lymphadenopathy

---

Staging of squamous carcinoma of the penis (Jackson)
- **I** – tumour confined to glans or prepuce
- **II** – invasion into shaft and corpora; no nodal or distal metastases
- **III** – tumour confined to penis; operable inguinal nodal metastases
- **IV** – tumours involves adjacent structures; inoperable inguinal lymph nodes and/or distant metastases

---

Treatment of penile carcinoma

- Primary lesions
  - Excision, partial amputation with a 2 cm resection margin
  - If amputation leaves an inadequate penile stump, consider a total penectomy with perineal urethrostomy
  - Can irradiate stage I with moulded iridium–192. Of irradiated stage II disease, 70% subsequently requires amputation
- Inguinal lymph nodes – 25–50% of patients present with palpable nodes but up to two-thirds of these are tumour-free on histology. Therefore treat for 6 weeks with antibiotics after excision and try to identify those with true metastases, which can then be irradiated or excised.

CLASSIFICATION OF MALE ERECTILE DYSFUNCTION (IMPOTENCE[6])

- Physical conditions
  - Painful conditions
    - Phimosis
    - Short frenulum
    - Peyronie's disease
  - Erectile dysfunction
    - Peyronie's disease
    - Chordee
    - Congenital causes, e.g. micropenis
- Functional causes
- Organic causes
  - Vascular
  - Neurological
  - Endocrine
  - Drug-induced
- Systemic disease

COMMON CAUSES AND TREATMENT OF ERECTILE FAILURE[18]

- Cause – Treatment
- Drugs – withdraw
- Vascular (arteriopathy or venous leak) – Caverjet, ligation of dorsal vein, sildenafil (Viagra)
- Diabetes – Caverjet, viagra
- Hormonal – hormonal replacement
- Neurologial, pelvic nerve and spinal cord disease – Caverjet, Viagra
- Pelvic surgery – Caverjet, Viagra

COMMON CAUSES OF PRIAPISM[4]

- Drugs, e.g. self injection therapy for impotence
- Idiopathic (no obvious predisposing cause)
- Spinal trauma
- Spinal neoplasm
- Sickle cell disease and coagulopathies
- Treatment – exercise, corporal aspiration (and irrigation), injection of α-agonists and surgical shunting

CAUSES OF GENITAL ULCERS[5]

- Diagnosis – clinical features
- Syphilis – firm, indurated painless ulcer
- Granuloma inguinale – rolled, elevated ulcer edge
- Chancroid – punched-out ulcer
- Genital herpes – group of vesicles/ulcers on a red base
- Traumatic ulcer – onset immediately after sexual activity
- Fixed drug eruption – specific drug ingestion
- Squamous carcinoma – raised often infected ulcer

SCROTUM AND TESTIS

CAUSES OF LUMPS IN THE GROIN[10]

Groin

- Above the inguinal ligament
  - Sebaceous cyst
  - Lipoma
  - Direct inguinal hernia
  - Indirect inguinal hernia
  - Imperfectly descended testis
  - Lipoma of the cord
  - Hydrocoele of the cord (rare)
  - Hydrocoele of the canal of Nuck (rare)
- Below the inguinal ligament
  - Sebaceous cyst
  - Lipoma
  - Femoral hernia
  - Lymph nodes
  - Saphena varix
  - Femoral artery aneurysm (true or false)
  - Ectopic testis
  - Neuroma of the femoral nerve (rare)
- Synovioma of the hip joint (rare)
- Obturator hernia (rare)

Scrotum

- Sebaceous cyst
- Indirect inguinal hernia
- Hydrocoele
- Epididymal cyst (spermatocoele)
- Epididymo-orchitis
- Testicular tumour
- Torsion of the testis
- Varicocoele
- Haematoceole
- Sperm granuloma
- Torsion of testicular appendage

CAUSES OF A SCROTAL SWELLING[2]

Structure	Pathology
Scrotal wall	Blood, haematuria Urinary extravasation Oedema from cardiac, hepatic or renal failure
Testis	Orchitis (mumps) Carcinoma Torsion of testis or appendix (see 6.1363) (hydatid of Morgagni)
Epididymis	Epididymitis Cyst Tumour Torsion of appendix epididymis TB
Spermatic cord	Hydroceole surrounding testis or involving cord only
Primary	Idiopathic
Secondary	Trauma, epididymo-orchitis, tumour, lymphatic obstruction Haematocoele Hernia Varicocele Lipoma

A PLAN FOR THE DIAGNOSIS OF SCROTAL SWELLINGS[12]

- Can you get above the swelling?
- Can you identify the testis and epididymis?
- Is the swelling translucent?
- Is the swelling tender?

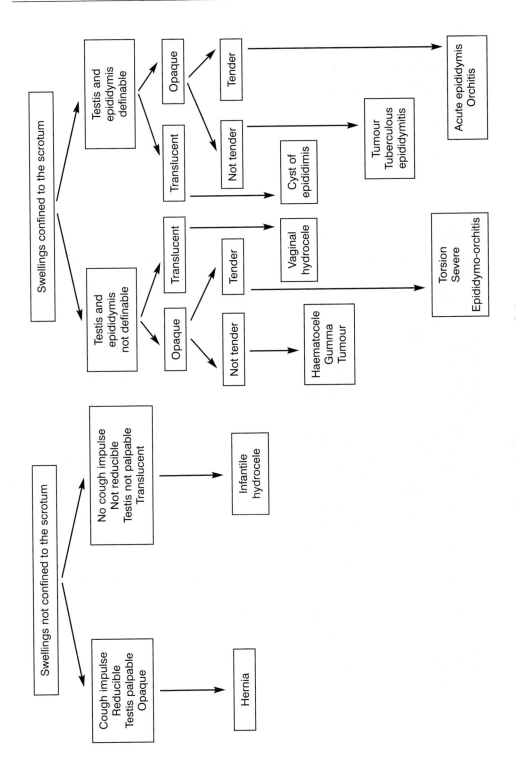

DIFFERENTIAL DIAGNOSIS OF SCROTAL DISCOMFORT AND SOLID MASS LESION[4]

	Torsion	Epididymitis	Tumour
History			
Age	Birth–20 years	Puberty-old age	15–35 years
Pain			
Onset	Sudden	Rapid	Gradual
Degree	Severe	Increasing severity	Mild or absent
Nausea			
Vomiting	Yes	No	No
Examination			
Testis	Swollen	Normal early	Mass
Epididymis	together and both tender	Swollen, tender	Normal
Spermatic cord	Shortened, thickened, often tender	Normal	Normal
Manual scrotal elevation	Pain constant	Pain decreased	Mild pain constant
Testicular position	Elevated	Normal	Normal
Opposite testis	Bell clapper	Normal	Normal
Observations			
Pyrexia	Absent	Often present	Absent
Urinalysis	Normal	Often infected	Normal

Treatment

- In torsion, the testis twist away from the median raphe. Attempts to untwist towards the raphe can be made whilst awaiting operation.
- After 7 h the seminiferous tubules are damaged though the Leydig cells which produce androgens are relatively spared.
- At operation the contralateral testis should also be fixed. If the testis is torted, ischaemic and unsalvagable it should be removed as it is thought that antibodies may be formed which will decrease the fertility in the normal testis.

TESTICULAR CARCINOMA[2]

Histological types	Incidence	Peak age incidence (years)
Seminoma	40%	30–40
Teratoma	32%	20–30
Mixed seminoma/teratoma	14%	25–35
Other tumours	7%	
Interstitial (Leydig tumour)		
Sertoli cell mesenchymal		
Gonadoblastoma		
Yolk sac tumour		
Mesothelioma		
Lymphoma		

Symptoms and signs

- Swelling of the testis usually painless, heaviness in the scrotum, palpable abdominal mass, spread to para-aortic lymph nodes or to left supraclavicular node, chest symptoms from a lung metastases

Investigations

- USS testis, tumour markers AFP, bHCG, LDH, CXR, CT scan

Tumour markers

- α-feto protein expressed by 70% of tumours
- Human chorionic gonadotrophin (HCG)expressed by 60% of tumours
- Lactate dehydrogenase

Note: 90% of teratomas produce one or more of these. All choriocarcinomas secrete HCG, <10% of seminomas secrete HCG whereas none produce AFP

Grading of teratomas

- Primary tumour histology
- Lymphatic invasion
- Vascular invasion – each increase the risk from 20 to 50%
- Presence of undifferentiated cells
- Absence of yolk sac elements

Staging of testicular tumours (after Peckham *et al*. 1979)[6]

- **Stage I** – confined to the testicle
- **Stage II** – involving nodes below the diaphragm (retroperitoneal or inguinal): a, <2 cm; b, >2 cm; c, >5 cm
- **Stage III** – involving nodes above the diaphragm (outside the retroperitoneal
- **Stage IV** – extralymphatic: pulmonary (L) or hepatic metastases (H)

Note: this staging is more commonly used in the UK than the TNM system

Treatment of testicular tumours

Seminoma

- **Stage I** – orchidectomy and radiotherapy to the para-aortic lymph nodes
- **Stages II–IV** – orchidectomy and platinum-based chemotherapy (e.g. cisplatinum, see below). For residual masses consider retroperitoneal lymph node dissection (RPLND)

Teratoma

- **Stage I** – orchidectomy and surveillance (monthly markers, 3-monthly CT scan for 1 year then annually, 5% will relapse and need chemotherapy)
- **Stages II–IV** – platinum-based chemotherapy (e.g. cisplatinum in POMB, ACE or BEP combinations) and removal of masses >2 cm RPLND. Further chemotherapy is advised if active disease in lymph nodes

Note: sperm count usually recovers 1–1.5 years after the chemotherapy

Follow up

- For life (>15 years)
- Major centres produce a 95% cure rate. The most successful treatment of any solid tumour

MALE INFERTILITY

Semen analysis: minimal standards of adequacy[4,9]

- On at least two occasions:
  - Ejaculate volume – 1.5–5.0 ml
  - Sperm density – >20 million/ml
  - Motility – >60%
  - Forward progression >60% or >2 (scale 1–4)
  - Morphology – >60% normal

and:

- No significant sperm agglutination
- No significant pyospermia
- No hyperviscosity
- Presence of fructose

UROLOGICAL INVESTIGATIONS

URINARY FLOW RATE[2]

Normal values in urodynamics	Men	Women
• Normal flow rates		
• Young <55	20 ml/s	18 ml/s
• Old 55+	12 ml/s	15 ml/s
• Minimum volume needed to be representative 150–200 ml		
• Bladder should fill without any great rise in pressure (<10–15 cm water), i.e. good compliance		
• Should void with a detrusor pressure (<60–70 cm water)		

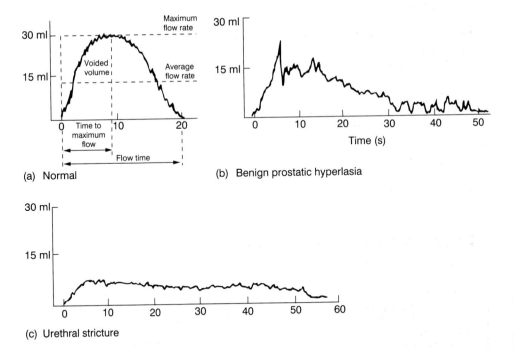

Figure 9.4 Characteristics of urinary free flow rate studies.

Static renal scan: DMSA

99m-technetium-labelled dimercaptosuccinic acid is taken up by the renal tubules and allows assessment of the size, position, parenchymal defects (scarring, cysts, tumours) and differential function.

Dynamic renal scan: DPTA or Mag3

99m-technetium-labelled diethylenetriamine pent-acetic acid is taken up by the kidney and excreted in the urine. There are three phases (see diagram):

- Vascular phase – isotope arrives at the kidney (normally lasts 30 s)
- Filtration phase – isotope concentrates in the kidney and passes into the collecting system
- Excretion phase – isotope is no longer arriving at the kidney but is being excreted

Renal artery stenosis causes impairment of vascular phase. Urinary tract obstruction prolongs the excretory phase (frusemide can be added to differentiate between obstruction or stasis.)

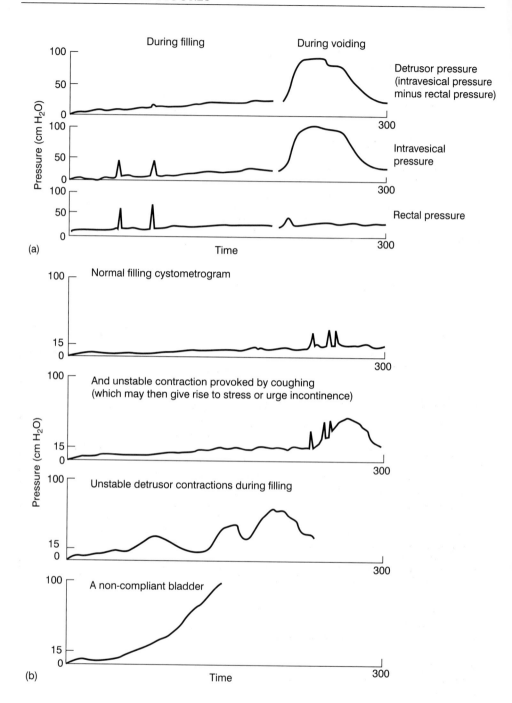

Figure 9.5 Normal and abnormal cystometrograms. Note: the peaks produced by coughing are subtracted out of the detrusor pressure. The detrusor pressure does not rise above 15 cm water during filling.

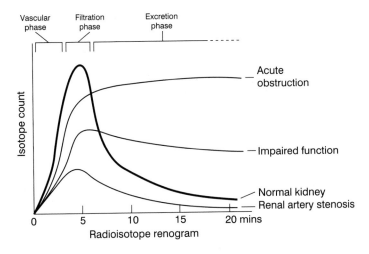

Figure 9.6 Normal and abnormal radioisotope renograms.

MAJOR INDICATIONS FOR AORTOGRAPHY AND RENAL ARTERIOGRAPHY[1]

Indication	Abnormality sought
Hypertension	
Suspected renal artery stenosis	Stenosis, post-stenotic dilatation
Suspected renin secreting tumour	Tumour circulation
Space-occupying lesion of the kidney	Tumour circulation
Acute renal failure	Suspected renal artery thrombosis or embolism arterial occlusion
Suspected polyarteritis nodosa	Arterial aneurysm
Loin pain, haematuria syndrome	Small arterial occlusion
Renal trauma	Bleeding point
Severe bleeding	Bleeding point
Proposed partial nephrectomy or	Renal circulation/anatomy
Anatrophic nephrolithotomy	Renal circulation anatomy
Proposed live donation of kidney graft	

10

PAEDIATRIC SURGERY

COMMON CLINICAL PROBLEMS OF LOW BIRTH WEIGHT BABIES[9]

- Preterm (<37 weeks)
- Surfactant deficiency
- Impaired temperature control
- Apnoeic attacks
- Jaundice
- Immature sucking or swallowing
- Hypocalcaemia
- Functional intestinal flow
- Infection
- Periventricular haemorrhage/ischaemia
- Necrotizing enterocolitis
- Patent ductus arteriosus

– small for gestational age (<10%)
– intrauterine death
– congenital malformation
– birth asphyxia
– meconium aspiration
– persistent pulmonary hypertension
– impaired temperature control
– hypoglycaemia
– polycythaemia

MECHANISMS OF HEAT LOSS IN NEWBORN BABIES AND STANDARD PROCEDURES TO CONSERVE HEAT[9]

Causes of heat loss	Methods of prevention
Evaporation of water from skin	Dry with warm towels Maintain high relative humidity
Convection through moving air	Avoid draughts Cloth babies in incubators
Conduction from skin to cold or wet surfaces	Prewarm all surfaces and bedding Clothe body and head
Radiation to cold room surface via cold air	Maintain high ambient room temperatures (24–26°C) Cover baby with plastic sheet and use woollen bonnet

STANDARD FLUID INTAKE OF TERM AND PRETERM BABIES (ML/KG/DAY)[9]

Day	Term	Preterm*
1	40	60
2	60	90
3	80	120
4	100	150
5	120	160
6	140	170
7	160	180
8	180	180

*If a preterm baby is nursed under a radiant warmer add an extra 40 ml/kg day but in those of very low and extremely low birth weight the total volume may need to be restricted to 75% to avoid a symptomatic patent ductus arteriosus. After 7 days the volume may need to be increased further if weight gain is unsatisfactory. Note: 100 mg/kg/day = 4 ml/kg/h.

CALCULATION OF FLUID REQUIREMENTS OF CHILDREN[14]

Weight (kg)	Water requirements
0–10	100 ml/kg/day, e.g. 10 kg = 1000 ml/day
10–20	1000 ml + 50 ml/kg/day for each kg >10, e.g. 15 kg = 1250 ml/day
>20	1500 ml + 25 ml/kg/day for each kg >20

Normal values for neonates and infants

- Serum osmolality – 20–260 mOsm/kg
- Urine osmolality
  - Neonate up to 450 mOsm/kg
  - Infant up to 700 mOsm/kg
  - Adult up to 1200 mOsm/kg
- Urine volume – <2500 g, 50–100 ml/kg/day
- >2500 g, 25 ml/kg/day

Postoperative fluid requirements

- Day 1 – 1/3 fluid requirements
- Day 2 – 2/3 fluid requirements
- Day 3 – full requirements

Note: young children have more severe stress response than adults therefore need to restrict fluids. To raise haemoglobin (Hb) by 1 g/dl needs 8 ml/kg blood or 5 ml/kg packed cells, or volume packed cells + weight × 3 × desired rise in Hb. For resuscitation of a shocked baby use HAS 4.5%.

Significant signs and symptoms likely to alert the medical personnel to underlying serious congenital abnormality[5]

- Material hydramnios (poly or oligo)
- Rapid respiration (>50/min)
- Respiratory distress (retraction, etc.)
- Cyanosis (a single episode)
- Excess salivation\abdominal distension
- Abdominal mass
- Vomiting of bile
- Failure to evacuate meconium (within 24 h)
- Inability to void (or inadequate or intermittent stream)
- Convulsions
- Lethargy (poor feeding)
- Jaundice (first 24 h)

MAJOR CONGENITAL ABNORMALITIES ENCOUNTERED[5]

- Symptoms – possible anomaly
- Respiratory – congenital heart disease
  - Cyanosis – congenital diaphragmatic disease
  - Breathlessness – oesophageal atresia and tracheo-oesophageal fistula

- Intestinal obstruction – atresia of small and large bowel
  - Vomiting, bile – stenosis: pylorus, small and large bowel
  - Distension – malrotation
  - Constipation
    - Meconium ileus
    - Meconium peritonitis
    - Hirschsprung's disease
    - Ano-rectal anomalies
    - Neonatal necrotizing enterocolitis
- Abdominal enlargement
  - Kidney
    - Polymulticystic kidneys
    - Hydronephrosis
    - Wilms's tumour
  - Liver
    - Tumour or cyst
    - Choledochal cyst
    - Ascites
    - Hydrometrocolpos
- Obvious defects
  - Cleft lip and palate
  - Cystic hygroma
  - Myelomeningocele
  - Sacrococcygeal teratoma
  - Exstrophy of bladder
  - Hypospadias
- Umbilical defects
  - Exomphalos, gastroschisis
  - Vitello-intestinal duct remnants
  - Urachal fistula
- Jaundice
  - Physiological
  - Neonatal hepatitis
  - Biliary atresia

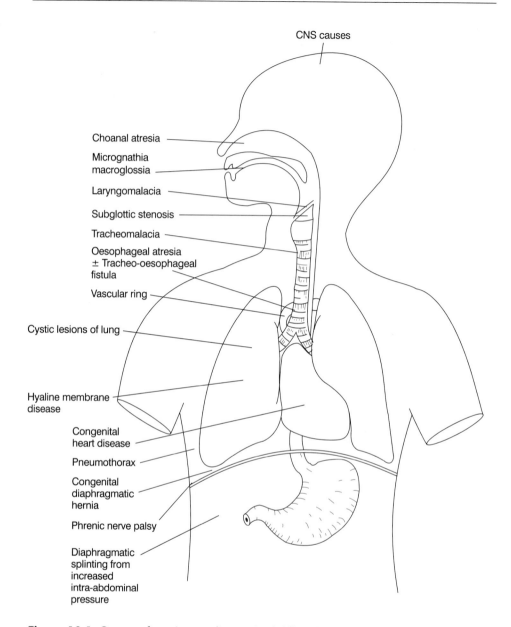

CNS causes

Choanal atresia

Micrognathia
macroglossia

Laryngomalacia

Subglottic stenosis

Tracheomalacia

Oesophageal atresia
± Tracheo-oesophageal
fistula

Vascular ring

Cystic lesions of lung

Hyaline membrane
disease

Congenital
heart disease

Pneumothorax

Congenital
diaphragmatic
hernia

Phrenic nerve palsy

Diaphragmatic
splinting from
increased
intra-abdominal
pressure

Figure 10.1 Causes of respiratory distress in childhood. From: *Fundamentals of Surgical Practice*; Greenwich Medical Media, 1998: page 546.

Oesophageal atresia and tracheo-oesophageal malformations

An endocardial cushion defect (1 in 3500) often part of the VACTERL (see Fig 10.2) complex (vertebral and anal defects, cardiac tracheo-oesophageal fistula, radial limb dysplasia, renal and radial limb abnormalities).

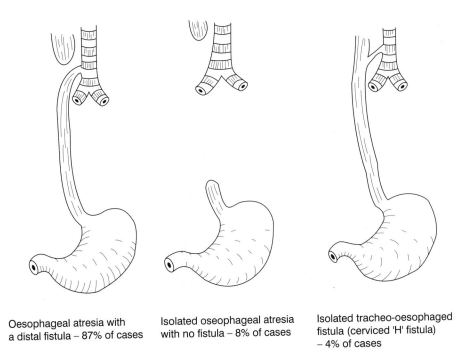

Oesophageal atresia with
a distal fistula – 87% of cases

Isolated oseophageal atresia
with no fistula – 8% of cases

Isolated tracheo-oesophaged
fistula (cerviced 'H' fistula)
– 4% of cases

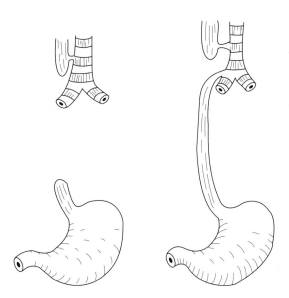

Figure 10.2 Types of oesophageal atresia and tracheo-oesophageal atresia. From: *Fundamentals of Surgical Practice*; Greenwich Medical Media, 1998: page 547.

Treatment

- Preoperatively decompress the proximal pouch with a stump tube on constant suction. Nurse in upright position. Perform gastrotomy if repair is to be delayed. Stretch proximal pouch daily in a pure atresia.
- Primary repair is undertaken if defect is <2 cm and no pneumonitis is present. Close fistula before the oesphagostomy is performed.
- Perform a delayed repair if the defect is >2 cm or >2.5 vertebral bodies in length.

Prognosis

- If weight >2500 g, no associated anomalies and no pneumonitis (100% survival).
- If either the weight 1800–2500 g, or have mild pneumonitis or a non-life-threatening anomaly (80% survival).
- If either the weight <1800 g, severe pneumonitis, severe life threatening anomaly (43% survival).

Follow up

- Well-recognized problems include: oesophageal dysmotility, dilated proximal pouch, gastro-oesophageal reflux, anastomotic stricture, recurrent fistula.

Malrotation of the intestine

- An abnormal placement and fixation of the midgut in the peritoneal cavity. It involves all the small intestine from the ampulla of Vater to the proximal 2/3 of the transverse colon. It can occur independently or be associated with diaphragmatic hernia, omphalcoele and gastroschisis.
- Normally, the midgut develops extra-abdominally and undergoes a 270° rotation when it migrates intraperitoneally. In malrotation, the caecum (and thus the appendix) is not in the right lower quadrant. The duodenum does not pass posteriorly to the superior mesenteric artery (SMA). The base of the small bowel is not fixed from the ligament of Treitz to the caecum but is anchored on the superior mesenteric artery. The caecum is usually fixed in the right upper quadrant by fibrous tissue (Ladd's bands) crossing the second portion of the duodenum.

Clinical problems

- Intestinal obstruction bilious vomiting.
- Midgut volvulus twisting on the vascular pedicle (SMA) causes ischaemia of the entire midgut.

Treatment

- Simple release of bands (Ladd procedure), mobilize the duodenum. Prevent obstruction or rotation by placing the caecum in left upper quadrant and the duodenum in right lateral.
- Perform an appendicectomy. Examine for associated abnormalities (e.g. duodenal web).
- If a volvulus is present, detort counterclockwise, resect gangrenous bowel (note: if large areas are necrotic do not resect but perform second look laparotomy in 24 h), perform a Ladd's procedure.

Prognosis

- Is related to the extent of bowel resection. Note: midgut volvulus reoccurs in 10%.

Gastroschisis and exomphalos

Gastroschisis and exomphalos are two types of abdominal wall defects.

- *Gastroschisis* is an opening in the abdominal wall adjacent to the umbilicus. The abdominal wall is completely formed but the peritoneal cavity does not enlarge enough to hold the abdominal contents.
  The protruding viscera (usually midportion of the small intestine, spleen, stomach, colon, occasionally liver) has no peritoneal covering and the intestine is therefore leathery and matted as a result of chemical peritonitis. Intestinal atresia is associated in 10% of cases.
- *Omphalocoele* is an opening in the abdominal wall at the umbilicus and is due to incomplete closure of the somatic folds of the anterior abdominal wall. The liver and small bowel most commonly protrude but as they are covered by a sac no signs of chemical peritonitis are present. If the caudal folds are included extrosphy of the bladder or cloaca can occur. Fifty percent of these infants have associate cardiac, neurological or genitourinary abnormalities, trisomy[13,18] and Beckwith–Weidman syndrome. It may form part of the Pentalogy of Cantell, which includes diaphragmatic hernia, cleft sternum, absent pericardium and intracardiac defects.
- Prenatal diagnosis is by ultrasound
- Preoperative management includes:
  - Gastrointestinal decompression, resuscitation, antibiotics, albumin for hypoproteinaemia.
  - Wrapping of abdominal contents in moist antibiotic soaked gauze. Placing the infant with gastroschisis on the side may prevent vascular compromise.
- Treatment – primary aim is to cover the abdominal viscera
  - *Gastroschisis* – if the closure is too tight the organs are covered temporarily with non-reactive silicon sheeting as a staged repair. Reduction should be completed in 10 days to avoid infection.
  - *Omphalocoele* – the defect may be closed in a staged manner, or with skin flaps allowing repair of the ventral hernia later or if there are associated abnormalities a granulating

(a)

(b)

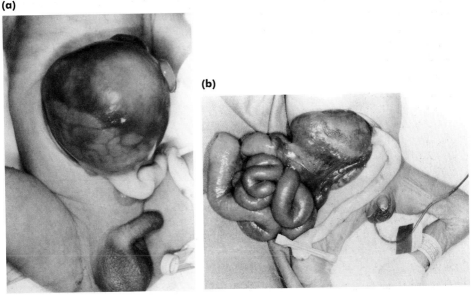

Figure 10.3 (a) Exomphalos (an umbilical defect) and (b) gastroschisis (a para-umbilical defect). From: *Fundamentals of Surgical Practice*; Greenwich Medical Media, 1998

eschar can be formed by coating the sac in silver sulphadiazine again repairing the ventral hernia later.

- Prognosis
  - Gastroschisis – mortality rate 5%, intestinal strictures can occur along with short bowel syndrome if gangrenous bowel excised.
  - Omphalocoele – mortality rate is 20–60%.

Pyloric stenosis

- A hypertrophy of the muscular layer of the pylorus causes gastric outlet obstruction leading to projectile non-bilious vomiting.
- Male:Female predominance of 4:1. Offspring of males affected have a four-fold risk of developing the condition, while offspring of females with pyloric stenosis have a 10-fold risk.
- Usually occurs in the first 2 weeks–2 months of life and leads to varying degrees of dehydration and hypochloraemic hypokalaemic metabolic alkalosis.
- Diagnosis – by palpating a mid-epigastric mass while the infant is feeding or by demonstrating on ultrasound that the pylorus is >15 mm and >4 mm wide. A string sign can be seen at the pylorus on contrast studies.
- Treatment
  - Nasogastric decompression. Monitor capillary acid/base balance.
  - Rehydrate over 12 h with 0.45% saline + 40 mM KCl/litre until bicarbonate <30 mmol/l.
  - Pyloromyotomy should not be undertaken until preoperative correction of alkalosis and volume deficit have brought the serum bicarbonate <28 mEq/ml. Feedings of glucose and water can be commenced 4 h postoperatively.

Note: giving extra potassium allows renal tubular exchange of K^+ for H^+. The preservation of H^+ allows correction of alkalosis.

Intussusception

- Has an incidence of 4/1000 – the majority present before 1 year of age.
- Most are ileocolic. Less than 10% have an identifiable anatomical source: a Meckel's diverticulum, a polyp, duplication cyst or ectopic pancreatic tissue.
- 90% are associated with lymphoid hyperplasia of Peyer's patches of the ileum.
- Diagnosis – colicky abdominal pain, drawing up of knees, 'red currant jelly' stool. Confirmed on ultrasound scan or barium enema, which may be therapeutic by hydrostatic reduction.
- Treatment – if hydrostatic reduction fails or peritonitis or perforation is present an operation is indicated. Reduction is achieved by squeezing the distal colon and pushing the intussuscepted bowel proximally. The proximal ileum should *not* be retracted. If reduction is impossible the area should be resected as should a precipitating anatomical lesion.

Hirschsprung's disease

- Congenital absence of the (incidence 1 in 5000) parasympathetic ganglia cells in the wall of the gastrointestinal tract. The affected portion of bowel is unable to relax or allow effective peristalsis.
- It always involves the rectum and can continue to involve the entire tract.
- Male predominance of 4:1. Of patients, 30% have an affected family member.
- Diagnosis – failure to pass meconium, constipation, abdominal distension, failure to thrive, enterocolitis.
  - Radiographs show a narrowed distal gut with a dilated proximal segment. Suction

biopsy is examined for Meissner's plexus in the submucosal layer. Full-thickness biopsy is examined for Auerbach's plexus in the muscular layer.

- Treatment – aim is to re-establish a functional, continent anus.
  - If functionally obstructed, can perform a colostomy using healthy tissue:
    - *Swenson* – normal bowel is sutured to a 1-cm cuff of the anomucocutaneous margin that is left once the affected bowel has been excised.

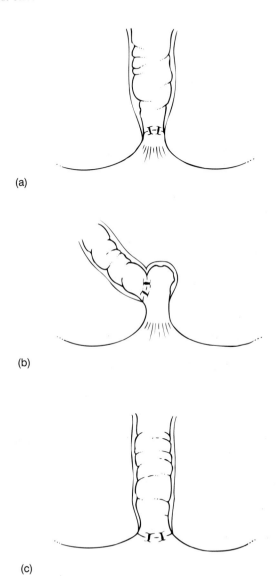

(a)

(b)

(c)

Figure 10.4 Operations for Hirsprung's disease. (a) Swenson's low colorectal anastomosis; (b) Duhamel's posterior colorectal anastomosis; (c) Soave's endorectal pullthrough after excision of the rectal mucosa.

- *Duhamel* – abnormal bowel is excised at the level of the peritoneal reflection. Normal bowel is tunnelled between the sacrum and rectum, and anastomosed end to side to the anorectum.
- *Soave* – affected colon is again incised at the level of the peritoneal reflection, the mucosa is removed and normal bowel is pulled down through the stripped anorectal segment and sutured to the ano rectal junction.

Imperforate anus

- Incidence 1–3/5000 births, twice as common in males.
- Low type (infralevator) – the rectum passes through the puborectalis sling (more common in girls).
- High type (supralevator) – the rectum does not pass through the puborectalis sling (more common in boys).
- Associated defects – fistula tracts may open into the post urethra in boys (giving rise to UTI or hypochloreamic acidosis due to absorption of chloride by colonic mucosa) and to the vagina in girls.
- Genitourinary renal agenesis and dysplasia, hypospadias, epispadias, bladder exstrophy, vaginal atresia and cloacal exstrophy.
- Other – gastrointestinal tract 15% (e.g. gastro-oesophageal fistula), heart 7%, skeletal system 6% (hemivertebra, sacral agenesis and spina bifida.
- Diagnosis – infant is inverted, a coin is placed on the anal dimple and the end of infra colonic air visualized by a lateral plain radiograph. A line is drawn from the posterior portion of the symphysis pubis to the tip of the coccyx (the pubococcygeal line) to give the position of the puborectalis sling and to assess which type of imperforation is present. If the distance from the tip of the colonic air to the anal dimple is >2 cm the lesion is supra levator. Air visible in the bladder suggests a posterior urethral fistulas and a supra levator type.
- Treatment – goal is a socially accepted, continent child:
  - *Infralevator* – if a fistula is present it can be dilated or relocated (Pott anal transfer) or opened with a Denis Brown cutback.
  - *Supralevator* – formation of a colostomy followed by formation of a neorectum at 1 year of age using the sagittal posterior anoplasty (Pena procedure).

Necrotizing enterocolitis

- Incidence 0.2–1/1000 – aetiology unknown. Theories include bacteria infection, hypoxia, umbilical artery catheterization, aortic thrombosis and hyperosmolar feeds have all been implicated. An ischaemic or hypoxic insult causes mucosal sloughing leading to bacterial invasion and intestinal gangrene and perforation. Usually occurs in the first few weeks of life in premature or low birth weight babies. Associated problems include premature rupture of membranes, prolonged labour, umbilical artery catheterization, respiratory distress, apnoea, resuscitation, low blood flow syndromes.
- Diagnosis – abdominal distension with bloody stools. Abdominal radiographs show distended bowel, oedematous intestines, a persistent distended loop, intramural gas (pneumatosis intestinalis) portal vein gas or intraperitoneal air.
- Treatment
  - Medical – gastrointestinal decompression, parenteral antibiotics, fluid resuscitation and nutritional support.
  - Surgical – if perforation occurs the involved intestine is resected with formation of a stoma. Relative indications for surgery include increasing peritonitis, failure to stabilize after 12 h of optimal medical management, a persistent loop or abdominal mass.

- Prognosis
  - Mortality rate 20% in those who require medical management; 50% in those requiring surgical management.
  - Strictures with subsequent abdominal obstruction occur in 30% of cases usually 3–6 weeks after the acute episode.

CAUSES OF SMALL BOWEL OBSTRUCTION IN CHILDREN[9]

- Small bowel atresia or stenosis
- Meconium ileus
- Hernia (internal or external)
- Volvulus (usually associated with malrotation)
- Duplication cyst
- Intussusception
- Intestinal aganglionosis
- Inspissated milk curd syndrome

CAUSES OF LARGE BOWEL OBSTRUCTION IN CHILDREN[9]

- Hirschsprung's disease
- Anorectal atresia or stenosis
- Meconium plug syndrome
- Colonic atresia or stenosis
- Extrinsic compression by cysts or tumours

CAUSES OF ABDOMINAL MASSES IN CHILDREN

- Gastrointestinal
  - Congenital pyloric stenosis
  - Crohn's disease
  - Constipation(faecal mass)
  - Intussusception
- Hepatopancreaticobiliary
- Liver
  - Biliary atresia
  - Portal hypertension
  - Metastases
  - Hepatitis
  - Hepatoblastoma
- Bile duct – choledochal cyst
- Pancreas – pseudocyst (traumatic)
- Genitourinary
  - Hydronephrosis
  - Nephroblastoma (Wilms')
  - Bladder (urethral valves)
  - Ovarian tumour or cyst

- Other
  - Neuroblastoma
  - Splenomegaly
  - Retroperitoneal sarcoma
  - Teratoma

CAUSES OF ABDOMINAL TUMOURS IN CHILDHOOD[4]

- Malignant abdominal tumours
  - Rhabdomyosarcoma
  - Renal – Wilms' tumour, renal cell carcinoma
  - Neuroblastoma
  - Hepatoblastoma
  - Lymphoma, lymphosarcoma
- Benign abdominal masses
  - Renal – renal abscess, multicystic dysplastic kidney, hydronephrosis, polycystic kidney, congenital mesoblastic nephroma
  - Mesenteric cysts
  - Choledochal cysts
  - Intestinal duplication cysts
  - Splenomegaly

RELATIVE FREQUENCY OF CHILDHOOD CANCERS[7]

- Leukaemia – 30%
- Tumours of central nervous system – 15%
- Bones and soft tissue tumours – 14%
- Lymphoma – 10%
- Neuroblastoma – 7%
- Wilms' tumour – 6–12%
- Retinoblastoma – 3%
- Others – 15%

Rhabdomyosarcomas

- Most common soft tissue tumour in childhood incidence peak at 1–7 years and adolescence
- Treatment
  - Multimodal chemotherapy, surgery and radiotherapy
  - Primary tumour together with affected lymph nodes is excised (taking into account resultant function and cosmesis)
  - Preoperative chemotherapy may reduce extent of surgery. Re-excision is undertaken if the initial resection is inadequate
  - Postoperative chemotherapy may eradicate residual disease and micrometastases (a combination of cyclophosphamide, vincristine, actinomycin D and adriamycin)
  - Local radiotherapy is given to residual disease and involved lymph nodes whereas chemotherapy is primary treatment if metastases at presentation
- Prognosis
  - Overall 2YS – 65%
  - 5YS
    - Group I – 90%

- Group II – 90%
- Group II – 64%
- Group IV – 30%
- With tumours of the genitourinary system and orbit have best prognosis. Unfavourable histology and tumours of the extremities, trunk and mucosa (perineum, retroperitoneum, abdominal viscera) have worse prognosis.

Neuroblastoma

- A neoplasm of adrenal and neural crest origin
- Incidence 1/10,000 live births. 50–60% present before 2 years of age. 65% arise in adrenal or non-adrenal retroperitoneal sites
- Rx – surgical excision in localized disease. Multidrug chemotherapy and radiotherapy in advanced disease
- Prognosis
  - Overall 3YS – 30–50%
  - Stage I – 100%
  - Stage II – 82%
  - Stage III – 42%
  - Stage IV – 30%
  - Poor prognostic factors high stage, unfavourable histology
- In general the older the child at diagnosis the worse the prognosis
- Two-year-olds have a 2YS rate of 77%; older children have only a 38% survival rate
- Primary abdominal lesion

Nephroblastoma (Wilms' tumour)

- An embryonoma of the renal parenchyma
- Incidence 7.8 per million of the population
- Peak incidence 3 years of age (80% present before 5 years of age)
- Affects both sexes equally
- Left kidney is 1.3 times more commonly affected than right
- Bilateral in 5.7% of cases

TNM pretreatment clinical classification of Nephroblastoma[7.523]

T – primary tumour
Tx – primary tumour cannot be assessed
T0 – no evidence of primary tumour
T1 – unilateral tumour $\leq$ 80 cm^2 (including kidney)★
T2 – unilateral tumour >80 cm^2 (including kidney)
T3 – unilateral tumour rupture before treatment
T4 – bilateral tumours
N – regional lymph nodes
Nx – regional lymph nodes cannot be assessed
N0 – no regional lymph node metastasis
N1 – regional lymph node metastasis
M – distant metastasis

★Area is calculated by multiplying the vertical and horizontal dimensions of the radiological shadow of the tumour and kidney.

National Wilms' Tumour Study staging system (NWTS–3)[9.2088]

I – tumour limited to kidney and completely excised
II – tumour extends beyond kidney but is completely excised
III – residual non-haematogenous tumour confined to abdomen (lymph-node involvement, diffuse tumour spillage, peritoneal implants, incomplete resection) unresectable
IV – haematogenous metastasis (liver, lung, bone, brain)
V – bilateral renal involvement at diagnosis (10% of cases)

Recommended treatment of Nephroblastoma[9.2089]

- Favourable histology
- **Stage I** – surgery and chemotherapy for 10 weeks to 6 months
- **Stage II** – surgery and chemotherapy for 18 months
- **Stage III** – surgery and radiotherapy (10–20 Gy) and chemotherapy for 15 months
- Unfavourable histology (any stage) and all stage IV
- Surgery and radiotherapy (20 Gy) and chemotherapy for 18 months

Prognosis[9]

- Overall survival – 90%
- With favourable histology 4YS
  Stage I – 97%
  Stage II – 95%
  Stage III – 91%
  Stage IV – 87%
- With unfavourable histology 4YS
  Stage I–III – 68%
  Stage IV – 58%
- Poor prognosis linked to:
  - Unfavourable histology, e.g. anaplasia or sarcomatous change
  - Advanced stage
  - Age >2 years (in general the older the child at diagnosis the worse the prognosis)
- Follow up – indefinite

Abnormalities of the testis and groin

- Undescended testes (maldescended) – a testis than has not descended into the scrotum by 1 year of age seldom descends spontaneously. An undescended testis has a 5-fold risk of becoming malignant even after orchidopexy. A testis should be brought into the scrotum soon after 12 months and before 2 years.
- Ectopic testis (malpositioned) – does not follow the normal path of descent.
- Undescended testis
  - Incidence
    - Preterm – 30% in those born at 30 weeks
    - Term – 4%
    - 1 year – 0.8–1.6%
  - Impalpable
    - Intra-abdominal – 33%
    - Vanishing – 33%
    - Intracanalicular – 33%
  - Palpable
    - Retractile – cremasteric reflex leads to movement to superficial inguinal pouch
    - Ectopic – 2%

- Maldescended – arrested in line of descent
- Age of orchidopexy <2 years
  - Indications
    - Malignancy (× 5)
    - Fertility (if fixed at 1–2 years of age leads to 80% fertility)
    - Cosmesis
    - Easy to spot later malignancy

SITES OF ECTOPIC TESTIS[8]

- Superficial inguinal ring
- Perineum
- Root of the penis
- Femoral triangle

Advantages of an early orchidopexy[2]
- May lessen the risk of malignancy and makes diagnosis easier
- Increases the chance of fertility
- Lessens the risk of torsion and makes the diagnosis easier
- Deals with the hernia
- Lessens the risk of trauma
- Reduces the psychological trauma

Defects of PPV

- Processus vaginalis usually closes at 36 weeks *in utero*. If it fails to close completely it leads to a hernia or hydrocele:
  - Hernia
    - <2 years of age – urgent, i.e. next operating list
    - Girls – 12% of all infant hernias, 75% bilateral
    - Boys – 60% right, 15% bilateral
    - If irreducible – sedation (i.m. pethidine +/– gallows traction) leads to reduction in 95%
  - Hydrocele
    - <2 years of age – expectant, i.e. leave until >2 years of age as it may resolve spontaneously
    - >2 years of age – routine surgery
  - Umbilical hernia
    - No operation required as minimal risk of strangulation only operate for cosmesis

CAUSES OF RECTAL BLEEDING IN CHILDHOOD[10]

- Fissure *in ano*
- Rectal polyps
- Rectal prolapse
- Meckel's diverticulum
- Intussusception
- Blood dyscrasia

LUMPS IN THE NECK IN CHILDHOOD[10]

- Anterior triangle
- Lymph nodes
- Primary infection – atypical mycobacterium, TB, toxoplasmosis
- Secondary infection – lymphadenitis
- Primary tumour – Hodgkin's, leukaemia
- Secondary tumour rare
- Thyroglossal cyst
- Dermoid cyst
- Goitre
- Submandibular gland
- Branchial cyst
- Posterior triangle
- Lymph nodes
- Cystic hygroma
- Sternomastoid tumour
- Parotid swelling

NEUROSURGERY

SIGNS OF NEUROSURGICAL DISEASE

FOCAL NEUROLOGY

- Frontal /parietal regions – speech plus motor function on dominant side
- Parietal/occipital regions – sensory plus spatial orientation
- Occipital – visual field
- Temporal – speech(dominant side) plus visual, epilepsy
- Cerebellum – coordination/balance
- Cranial nerves – I–XII

RAISED INTRACRANIAL PRESSURE (ICP)

- Normal <200 mmH$_2$O
  - Increased volume of CSF
    - Obstruction of normal flow in ventricles, obstructive hydrocephalus
    - Obstruction of normal flow in subarach space – communicating hydrocephalus
    - Excessive CSF production – papilloma of choroid plexus
  - Increased cranial contents
    - Space-occupying lesion
      - Tumour
      - Abscess
      - Cyst
      - Haematoma
  - Increased volume of intracranial blood
    - Venous obstruction of intracranial sinuses
    - Vasodilatation in hypercapnia
  - Decreased skull size – craniosynostosis

CLINICAL FEATURES OF RAISED ICP

- Headache, especially in the morning
- Vomiting
- Drowsiness
- Papilloedema plus retinal haemorrhages
- Fontanelle bulging in children

LATE SIGNS DUE TO DISTORTION OF BRAIN SHAPE

- Tentorial notch pressure
  - Ipsilateral
    - IIIrd nerve – dilated pupil
    - Pyramidal tract – motor weakness
- Posterior cerebral art – occipital lobe infarction> permanent homonymous hemianopia
  - Downward pressure on brainstem
    - Bilatera – VIth nerve
  - Cerebellar tonsillar herniation
    - Neck stiffness
    - Bradycardia, hypertension (Cushing response)
    - Respiratory arrest

MENINGEAL IRRITATION

Features

- Headache
- Neck stiffness
- Nausea, vomiting
- Photophobia

Causes (cf. peritonitis)

- Blood – subarachnoid haemorrhage
- Pus
  - Spontaneous
  - Post-head injury (especially damage to paranasal sinuses), pneumococcal meningitis
  - Dermoid fistula (midline lesion over vertex of skull)
- Malignant cells – primary or secondary
- Chemical
  - Post-LP
  - Cholesterol meningitis – leakage of cholesterol via dermoid, epidermoid cyst or craniopharyngioma

Investigations

- Skull XR
- CT scan
- MRI/MRA scans
- Angiography
- Lumbar puncture

BRAIN TUMOURS

PRIMARY OR SECONDARY

- Overall incidence 5/100,000
  - Neuroepithelial – 50%
  - Metastatic – 15%
  - Menigioma – 15%
  - Pituitary – 8%

Risk factors

- Non-firm genetic or environmental link established
- Increased incidence of tumours in:
  - Neurofibromatosis – glioma, meningioma, acoustic neuroma
  - Tuberous sclerosis – astrocytoma
  - Von Hippel–Lindau – haemangioblastoma

Extracerebral

- Meninges – meningiomas, pressure symptoms, good prognosis
- Nerves – neuroma (especially acoustic neuroma), tinnitus, vertigo, facial pain
- Vascular – haemangioblastoma (2%), cerebellum, highly vascular

- Pituitary – anterior, adenoma
  - Optic chiasm compression, bitemporal hemianopia
  - Pituitary function decreased, hypothyroid, adrenal, gonad
  - Secreting – prolacatin, corticotrophin or growth hormone
  - Bone – chordoma <1%, embryo notochord remnant

Intracerebral

- Gliomas – grade 1–4 depending on histology, rapid presentation, poor prognosis grade 4 (glioblastoma multiforme)
  - Astrocytoma
  - Oligodendroglioma
  - Ependymoma
  - Medulloblastoma
- Lymphoma
- Pineal gland tumour <1%
  - Parinaud syndrome(upward gaze ocular convergence paralyses)
  - Germinoma (80–90%), choricarcinoma, endodermal sinus tumour
  - Raised AFP, HCG
- Papilloma of choroid plexus
- Metastases

NON-MALIGNANT SPACE-OCCUPYING LESIONS

- Abscess
- Congenital cysts
- Parasitic cysts
- Granuloma, e.g. TB
- Vascular anomalies

Management principles

- Establish diagnosis
  - Treat raised ICP
  - Anti-convulsant therapy
  - Preoperative devascularization of tumours, e.g. large meningioma via embolization
  - Surgical tumour biopsy /removal
    - Stereotactic
    - Craniotomy
  - Adjuvant treatment – radiotherapy

METASTATIC TUMOURS

- Present in 30% of patients with systemic cancer
- Lesions in distal arterial fields, especially mid cerebral articulation
- Multiple
- Approximate primary origin
  - Lung – 40%
  - Melanoma – 11%
  - Kidney – 11%
  - Colon – 8%

CEREBRAL ABSCESS

- 75% local spread of infection – frontal sinus/middle ear
- 25% systemic spread, congenital heart lesion
- Treat with
  - Burr hole aspiration
  - Antibiotics
  - Other management as for tumour

HEAD INJURY

- Blunt
- Penetrating
- Cause of trauma, e.g. collapse, post-epilepsy
- Most common cause of death in children
- High morbidity post-major head injury

Damage to:

- Brain – acceleration–deceleration
  - Diffuse brain injury
    - Mild = concussion
    - Severe = dementia, spasticity
    - Pathological neuronal damage due to rotatory shear forces
  - Local brain injury
    - Contracoup damage
    - Localized intracerebral/subarachnoid bleeding and oedema
- Skull fractures
  - Linear
  - Basal
  - Compound
  - Depressed

Complications of head injury

- Intracranial bleed – extradural/subdural/subarachnoid/intracerebral
- Cerebral ischaemia
  - Respiratory failure
  - Circulatory failure
- Cranial nerve damage II, III, V–VIII
- CSF rhinhorea
- CSF otorrhoea
- Brain abscess
- Meningitis
- Epilepsy
- Diabetes insipidus
- Traumatic fat embolism (in major trauma)
- Carotico-cavernous fistula (rare)

Basic management of head injuries

Trauma protocol

- **A** – Airway assessment – intubate and ventilate in unable to maintain own airway
- **B/C** – Breathing/ventilation – respiratory rate, pulse, BP, O_2 saturation and resuscitate as appropriate
- **D** – Disability – conscious level (GCS), pupil size and reaction, peripheral neurology
- **E** – Exposure/environmental control – head, scalp, ear and nose examination

Further assessment

- Need to exclude intracranial bleed or serious brain injury

CT scan indications

- Skull fracture plus decreasing GCS/confusion/focal neurology/seizures
- Persistent confusion/decreased GCS
- Deteriorating conscious level
- Depressed skull fracture
- Penetrating/open skull fracture with CSF Leak
- Difficult assessment, e.g. alcohol

Skull X-ray indications

- Loss of consciousness/amnesia
- Suspected fracture
- CSF leak

Admission and observation indications

- Confused, decreased conscious level but stable
- Persistent headache, nausea, vomiting
- Difficult assessment
- Poor social support.

INTRACRANIAL BLEEDS

Extradural

- Damage to middle meningeal artery or large venous sinus
- Usually present within 24 h post-injury, occurs after lucid interval
- History of trauma
- Swelling +/– skull fracture over site
- Deteriorating conscious level – late signs – ipsilateral pupil dilation, contralateral motor weakness
- Need craniotomy and clot evacuation

Subdural

- Acute – post-trauma to frontal/temporal lobes, assigned with brain swelling, damage to bridging veins
- Chronic – infantile <6 months or elderly >60 years of age, cerebral atrophy, coagulopathy
- Decreased conscious level
- Meningeal irritation
- Need craniotomy and clot evacuation

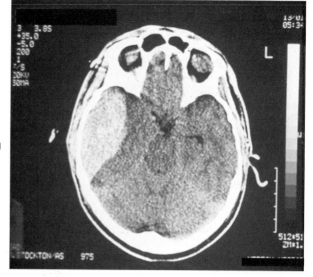

Figure 11.1 Axial CT showing a large right temporal extradural haematoma. The fresh blood is highly dense (white). From: *Sports Medicine: Problems and Practical Management* (Eds. E. Sherry & D. Bokor); Greenwich Medical Media, 1997: page 81.

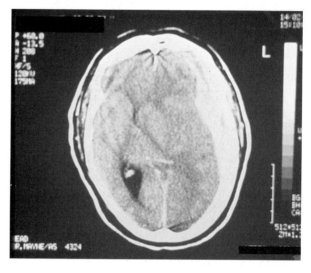

Figure 11.2 Axial CT of a subdural haematoma with midline shift. Note the haematoma is characteristically more extensive and crescenteric in shape. From: *Sports Medicine: Problems and Practical Management* (Eds. E. Sherry & D. Bokor); Greenwich Medical Media, 1997: page 81.

Subarachnoid

- Post-traumatic – severe head injury
- Spontaneous
  - Rupture of saccular intracranial aneurysm
  - Present in 3% of individuals, circle of Willis
  - Sudden onset headache
  - Meningism
  - Deteriorating conscious level
  - Focal neurological signs
- Complications

- Death in massive bleed
- Irreversible cerebral ischaemic damage
- Rebleed 4% in 24 h; 19% in 2 weeks
- Cerebrovascular vasospasm
- Hydrocephalus
- Electrolyte disturbance
- Cardiac arrhythmia

Diagnosis

- History
- Examination
- CT – presence of blood in subarachnoid space
- LP – xanthochromia

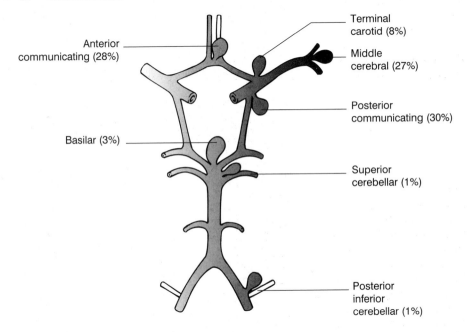

Figure 11.3 Anatomical distribution of cerebral aneurysms (figures denote percentage of total).

- MRA
- Angiography – identify possible site of lesion

Treatment

Medical

- Resuscitation – intubate and ventilate if required
- Anti-hypertensives – nimodipine, decreases risk of neurological deficit and death
- Anti-convulsants – phenytoin
- Raised ICP – steroids

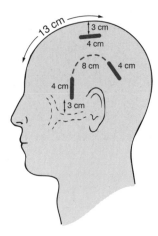

Figure 11.4 Sites of burr holes.

- Hypervolaemic haemodilution > reduces vasospasm and cerebral ischaemia

Surgical

- Venticulostomy in progressive hydrocephalus
  - Lesion identifies and ablated via craniotomy and clipping
  - Alternative technique; endovascular occlusion

CEREBRAL ANEURYSM

Incidental findings

- >10 mm high risk of rupture = elective treatment advised
- <5 mm, or difficult to approach surgically – monitor wCT scans

Infectious aneurysm

- Subacute endocarditis
- Antibiotics and monitoring

12

PLASTIC SURGERY

FUNCTIONAL ANATOMY OF THE SKIN – TERMINOLOGY[6]

- Cyst: a tumour that contains fluid
- Hamartoma: an overgrowth of one or more cell types that are normal constituents of the organ in which they arise. The commonest examples are haemangiomas, lymphangiomas and neurofibromas
- Macule – a flat impalpable lesion, e.g. a port wine stain
- Naevus – a lesion present from birth, composed of mature structures normally found in the skin but present in excess or in abnormal disposition. This type of lesion is also referred to as hamartoma. The term 'naevus' is also used to describe lesions composed of naevus cells as in melanocytic or pigmented naevi
- Papilloma – a benign overgrowth of epithelial tissue
- Papule – a small elevated lesion
- Plaque – an elevated area, usually >2 cm across
- Pustule – a raised lesion that contains pus
- Tumour – literally, a swelling. Commonly but inaccurately used to mean a malignant swelling
- Ulcer – an area of dissolution of an epithelial surface
- Vesicle – a small blister

PLASTIC SURGERY – TERMINOLOGY[6]

- Graft – a piece of tissue, usually skin, that is taken from one part of the body and transferred to a secondary site where it must establish a blood supply by the ingrowth of new vessels if it is to survive. It follows that grafts will not survive (take) on avascular surfaces such as infected or necrotic tissue, exposed cartilage, tendon or most cortical bone.
- Flap – tissue that remains attached to the body by a pedicle that carries the blood supply to the flap. Flaps do not need to establish a blood supply from the recipient bed for survival, and can be used to cover areas where a graft will not take.
- Contraction – a normal physiological healing process that occurs at the margin of a wound and decreases the final size of the wound; contraction usually benefits the surgeon by reducing the ultimate size of a defect.
- Contracture – the scar tissue that results from the process of contraction. Contracture may result in deformity across a joint that requires release with a skin graft or flap.
- Epithelialization – a process of migration of epithelial cells from a wound edge or adnexal structure to resurface the wound. Epithelialization over an area of full-thickness skin will not contain dermis and will therefore have a tendency to hypertrophy and instability.
- Granulation tissue – the tissue that forms in any open wound, where that epithelial surface has been lost. Granulation tissue is composed of fibroblasts, capillaries (neoendothelial loops) and macrophages.
- Donor defect – the site from which a graft or flap is taken.
- Recipient site – the site to which a graft or flap is transferred.

CLASSIFICATION OF CYSTS[8]

- Congenital
  - Sequestration dermoids
  - Tubuloembryonic (tubulodermoid)
  - Cysts of embryonic remnants

- Acquired
  - Retention
  - Distension
  - Exudation
  - Cystic tumours
  - Implantation dermoids
  - Trauma
  - Degeneration
- Parasitic – hydatid, trichiniasis, cysticercosis

BURNS

CLASSIFICATION OF BURNS[8]

Type of burn	Tissue injury
Heat injury	
• Scalds	Partial thickness/deep dermal loss
• Fat burns	Usually full thickness of skin loss
• Flame burns	Patches of full and partial thickness
• Electrical burns	Full thickness with deep extensions
Cold injury	
• Freezing injury	Ice formation – tissue freezing
• Frostbite	Direct damage and vasospasm
Friction burns	Heat plus abrasion
Physical damage	
Ionizing radiation	Early tissue necrosis, later tissue dysplastic changes
Chemical burn (acid or alkali)	Inflammation, tissue necrosis and allergic response

SELECTED CHARACTERISTICS SUGGESTING DEPTH OF INJURY OF BURNS[9]

- First-degree
  - Red, erythematous (superficial)
  - Very sensitive to touch
  - Very painful
  - Usually moist
  - No blisters
  - Surface markedly and widely blanches to light pressure
- Second-degree (partial skin thickness)
  - Erythematous or whitish with a fibrinous exudate
  - Wound base is sensitive to touch
  - Painful
  - Commonly have blisters
  - Surface may blanch to pressure

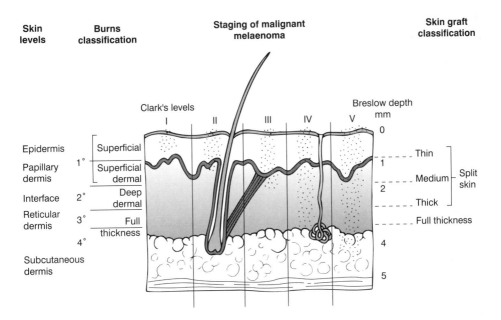

Figure 12.1 Skin depth related to malignant melanoma, burns and skin grafts.

- Third-degree (full skin thickness)
  - Surface may be:
    - White and pliable
    - Black, charred and leathery
    - Pale and mistaken for normal skin
    - Bright red from haemoglobin fixed in the subdermis
  - Generally anaesthetic or hypoaesthetic
  - Subdermal vessels do not blanch
  - No blisters
  - Hair easily pulled from the follicle
- Fourth-degree – involves deep tissues including fascia, muscle, bone, and tendons

CLASSICATION OF THERMAL BURNS[5]

	Major burn	Moderate burn	Minor burn
Size: partial thickness	>25% adults >20% children	15–25% adults 10–20% adults	<15% adults <10% children
Size: full thickness	>10%	2–10%	<2%
Primary areas involved (head, neck, hands, feet and perineum)	Major harm	Not involved	Not involved

	Major burn	Moderate burn	Minor burn
Inhalation injuries	Major burn if present or suspected	Not suspected	Not suspected
Associated injury Comorbid factors	Major burn if present Poor risk patients	Not present Relatively good risk patients	Not present Not present
Miscelleneous Treatment environment	Electrical injuries Specialised burn centre	General hospital designated team	Often managed as an outpatient

PRIMARY SURVEY OF BURNS PATIENT[9]

Activities necessary in the initial approach to a seriously injured patient:
- Provide an adequate airway with C-spine immobilization
- Provide sufficient breathing including intubation if necessary
- Evaluate circulation considering clinical signs and symptoms of shock and tamponade obvious bleeding
- Determine the presence of associated life-threatening conditions (e.g. obstructed airway, cardiac tamponade, tension pneumothorax, etc.)
- Initiate fluid resuscitation by large bore venous cannulae
- Remove jewellery and clothing
- Place urinary and nasogastric catheters
- Order appropriate radiographic and laboratory evaluations

SECONDARY SURVEY OF BURNS PATIENT[9]

Activities that follow the primary survey to evaluate the burned patient completely and to develop a treatment plan:
- Obtain a medical history
- Perform a head-to-toe physical examination
- Record a detailed burn diagram
- Administer analgesics intravenously
- Administer tetanus prophylaxis
- Cover wounds
- Evaluate and perform indicated escharotomies and fasciotomies
- Consider transfer to other facility if necessary

TRANSFER CONSIDERATIONS[9]

- Second- and third-degree burns >10% body surface area (BSA) in patients <10 or >50 years of age.
- Second- and third-degree burns >20% BSA in patients between 10 and 50 years of age.
- Second- and third-degree burns with a serious threat to functional and cosmetic impairment that involve the face, hands, feet, genitalia, perineum and other major joints.
- Third-degree burns >5% BSA.

- Specialized injuries such as electrical burns, including lightning and chemical burns, with serious threat to functional or cosmetic impairment.
- Significant inhalation injuries.
- Circumferential burns of the extremities or the chest.
- Pre-existing medical disorders that complicate management, prolong recovery or affect mortality.
- Paediatric patients in hospitals without qualified personnel or equipment for the care of children.
- Concomitant trauma in which the burn injury poses the greater risk of mortality; however, if the trauma poses the greater or immediate risk, the patient should receive treatment in the initial trauma centre.

INDICATIONS FOR ANTIBIOTICS IN BURN PATIENTS[9]

- Deterioration of the patient's overall clinical condition together with a substantial increase in the number of bacteria cultured from the wound (from scant or moderate growth to abundant growth).
- Signs or symptoms of bacteraemia with or without positive blood cultures.
- Less specific findings of sepsis such as isolated cardiovascular failure, altered mental alertness, hypothermia, spiking fevers or the onset of ileus.

BURN FORMULA[6]

- Estimation of percentage of the body surface burned to assess severity
- Adults – rule of nines
- Infants – head is 19% of the body surface and each lower extremity is 13%
- Prognosis: Percentage burn + age gives a rough estimate of the chance of dying as a result of the burn

THEORY OF FLUID REPLACEMENT AFTER A BURN (AFTER SETTLE)[6]

- A fluid containing salt and water is required for 48 h after a burn.
- Total volume is between 2 and 4 ml/kg/% body surface area burn and should contain 0.5 mmol sodium/kg/% burn.
- Total volume required can be reduced by the addition of colloid or by using hypertonic saline solutions.
- Water loss through a burn wound will vary according to the environment, but when nursed in conventional dressings, metabolic water requirements will be ~1.5–2 ml/kg/h, with a minimum 30 ml/h for infants.

Note: A burns' formula is only a guide to the average amount of fluid that can be required examples are shown in the following table.

CALCULATING FLUID REPLACEMENT FOR THE BURN (NOT INCLUDING OTHER INSENSIBLE LOSSES)

Muir and Barclay (the standard UK formula)

- Plasma – 0.5 ml/kg/% total body surface area (TBSA) of burn per period
- Albumin – 0.65 ml/kg/% TBSA of burn per period

- Periods are broken down into (36 h total)
  - 3×4 h
  - 2×6 h
  - 1×12 h

Baxter, Parkland formula

- In first 24 hours give: Lactated ringers – 4 ml/kg/% TBSA of burn
  - 50% of total volume in first 8 h
  - 50% of total volume in next 16 h
- In second 24 h – 2 litres 5% dextrose plus 0.5 ml/kg/% TBSA as colloid

METHODS OF CLOSING SKIN DEFECTS[22]

- Relaxing incisions
- Split skin grafts
- Whole thickness grafts
- Skin flaps
- Foreign skin (xenograft)
- Free flaps

INDICATIONS FOR SKIN GRAFTS[6,10]

- Burns
- Traumatic skin loss
- Ulcers and pressure sores
- Wide excisions of skin tumours
- Extensive ulcers
- Fasciotomy closure
- Flap donor defects
- As cover for large granulating wounds

TYPES OF SKIN GRAFT[15]

- Free
- Skin flaps
- Pedicled
- Free with microsurgical anastomosis

Free partial thickness (Thiersch)

- Use on
  - Large denuded areas
  - Granulating wounds
  - Site where contracture of the graft is of little cosmetic or functional consequence

Advantage – takes easily

Disadvantage – contractures are inversely proportional to the thickness of the graft

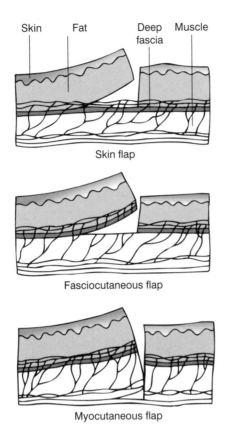

Figure 12.2 Classification of flaps according to anatomical component.

Free full thickness (Wolfe)

- Needs
  - Strict asepsis
  - Vascular recipient site
- Advantage – no contracture, therefore better cosmesis
- Disadvantage
  - No tolerance of sepsis
  - Closure of donor site
- No free graft will take on tendon, bone, joint surface or within a mucosal cavity

Factors in graft survival

- Skin applied to healthy granulating surface
- No subcutaneous fat transplanted
- Accurate apposition to granulating surface
- Immobilization of graft
- Revascularization within 48 h by capillary loops from granulation tissue
- Absence of infection (especially haemolytic *Streptococcus*)
- General health of patient

Reasons for graft failure

- Failure of revascularization
- Haematoma/seroma
- Poor immobilization
- Infection
- Poor recipient bed (bone, cartilage, tendon, etc.)

Technique of grafting

- Partial thickness using dermatome (free hand, power, drum)
- Full thickness matching donor and recipient site and using scalpel to dissect out donor site

SKIN FLAPS

- Indications
  - Poor recipient site
  - Good cosmesis necessary
- Specific sites
  - Eye lid
  - Cheek
  - Intracavity
  - Breast reconstruction
- Types
  - Cutaneous pattern flap
  - Axial
  - Musculocutaneous
  - Free with microsurgical anastomosis
  - Pedicled flap
- Disadvantages of pedicled flaps
  - May take several operations and months to remove a flap from a donor to a recipient site, whereas free grafting is performed at a single operation
  - May not match skin colour and hair

INDICATIONS FOR PEDICLE FLAPS[10]

- Wound closure in areas of poor vascularity, e.g. over ribs after extended mastectomy
- Area of bone where padding is needed, e.g. over sacrum or ischial tuberosity
- Facial reconstructive surgery

FREE GRAFTING WITH MICROSURGICAL ANASTOMOSIS OF VESSELS

Types of graft

- Cutaneous
- Myocutaneous
- Myo-osseocutaneous
- Osseocutaneous

Specific donor sites

- Type – vascular basis
- Iliofemoral – superficial circumflex iliac vessels

Flap circulation

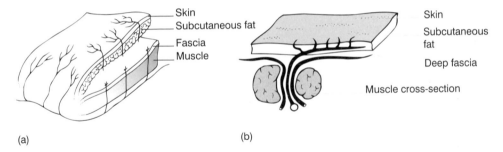

Skin
Subcutaneous fat
Fascia
Muscle

Skin

Subcutaneous fat

Deep fascia

Muscle cross-section

(a)   (b)

Figure 12.3 Flap circulation. (a) Random pattern flap. (b) Axial pattern flap. Flap elevation results in the interruption of the vertical musculocutaneous perforators, except for those at the base of the flap.

Flap configuration

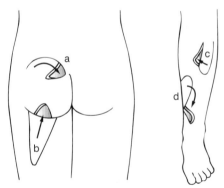

Figure 12.4 Flap configuration. (a) Rotation flap (semicircular); (b) Advancement flap (V-Y); (c) Transposition flap (rectangular); (d) Island flap.

- Radial forearm – radial artery
- Deltopectoral – anterior division of internal mammary vessels
- Scalp – superficial temporal vessels
- Thoracodorsal – lateral thoracic vessels
- Foot – dorsalis pedis and long saphenous vein
- Greater omentum – gastroepiploic vessels (for surface cover or filling cavity)

Technique
- Anastomosis needs two patient veins for every artery
- Very accurate apposition with no tension and interrupted sutures using 9/0 prolene
- Very gentle tissue handling and meticulous dissection using jewellers instruments

- Full heparinization of vessels
- Nerve anastomoses – excise all neuromata and use perineural sutures
- Use operating microscope unless the vessels are >2–3 mm in size, then use an operating loupe (× 2–4 magnification)

Problems

- Donor tissue is anaesthetic
- Graft failure due to:
  - Poor vascularity
  - Sutures under tension
  - Vessel kinking
  - Extrinsic pressure on vessels
  - Haematoma
  - Infection

Note: If failure is suspected then inject fluorescein intravenously and observe the graft under ultraviolet light for evidence of fluorescence suggesting vascular viability.

ASSESSMENT OF FREE FLAPS POSTOPERATIVELY[6]

Healthy flap	Arterial failure	Venous failure
Pink, normal colour	Pale–white–mottled	Red–blue–black
Normal refill	No refill	Rapid–instant refill
Normal turgor	Flaccid	Swollen, tense
Normal or elevated temperature	Cool–cold	Normal–cool
Normal bleeding	Absent bleeding	Blue–black ooze

SKIN CANCERS

BASAL CELL CARCINOMA[18]

- Incidence – 652/100,000 population
- Aetiology and associated factors
  - Ultraviolet light
  - Previous irradiation
  - Arsenical ointment
  - Xeroderma pigmentosum
  - Sebaceous naevus of Jadassohn
  - Hereditary multiple naevoid basal cell carcinoma syndrome (Gorlin and Goltz)
- Types
  - Nodular or solid – head and neck, shiny raised nodule with 'rolled' edges which ulcerates
  - Cystic – translucent
  - Pigmented – may be either nodular or cystic
  - Morphoeic – rolled edges are absent and often look like scars
  - Cicatrizing – slowly spreads peripherally leaving a central thin papery scar

Treatment

- Single lesions – excision (margin 2 or 5 mm in morpheic lesions) or radiotherapy (not used around the eye or overlying cartilage) produce cure rates of 95–98%
- Multiple – topical 5-fluorouracil

SQUAMOUS CELL CARCINOMA[18]

- Incidence – 160/100,000 population
- Tend to arise in previously damaged skin, i.e. after chronic solar damage in white skinned races or burns, the lips of pipe smokers and after exposure to industrial carcinogens such as arsenic, tar and oils

Treatment

- Excision (with a 10 mm margin) or radiotherapy in frail patients
- Full clearance of the draining lymphatic field is required if nodes are clinically involved

MALIGNANT MELANOMA[18]

- Incidence – 19/100,000 population is the least common skin cancer but it has the greatest malignant potential as it spreads early via the blood stream

Clinical features indicative of the development of a melanoma in a pre-existing mole[5]

- Change in size
- Change in outline – irregular
- Change in elevation – thicker, more palpable, nodules
- Change in colour – increasing pigmentation, depigmentation, irregular pigmentation
- Change in surrounding tissues – pigmented halo, satellite lesions
- Development of symptoms – itching, awareness of lesion, serious discharge and bleeding

Types of malignant melanoma

Type	Characteristics	Incidence	Prognosis
Superficial spreading	Initial horizontal growth. Prognosis worsens when growth phase becomes vertical	70%	Variable
Acral lentigenous	Palms, soles, subungal, retinal, genital.	13%	Poor
Nodular	Vertical growth	10%	Poor
Lentigo maligna	Flat, slow growing. Predominantly in facial areas of the elderly	7%	Good

EFFECT OF BRESLOW'S MICROSTAGING ON REGIONAL NODE METASTASES AND SURVIVAL[8]

Thickness of lesion	Incidence of nodal involvement	5-year survival	Recommended width of excision
< 0.75 mm	0	100%	2 mm (i.e. biopsy)
0.76–1.5 mm	10%	80–90%	20 mm
1.6–3.0 mm	20%	60%	50 mm
> 3.0 mm	40% or more	<50%	50 mm

CLARK'S HISTOLOGICAL STAGING AND PROGNOSIS[5]

Level of involvement	Histological node involvement (%)	5-year survival (%)
I – melanoma does not penetrate the basement membrane	0	100
II – melanoma extends into the papillary dermis	5	90–100
III – melanoma reaches the junction between the papillary and reticular dermis	10–30	80–90
IV – melanoma extends into the reticular dermis	30–40	60–70
V – melanoma extends into the subcutaneous fat	60–70	15–30

Treatment[18]

- Excision biopsy followed by wide local excision when necessary
- Life-long regular surveillance or self examination of regional gland field
- Surgical elimination of involved palpable gland where appropriate
- Radiotherapy is used in palliation and trials or adjuvant or late chemotherapy are in progress
- Immunotherapy may be possible in future

ULCERS

CAUSES OF CHRONIC ULCERATION[12]

- Infection
- Repeated trauma
- Anoxia, ischaemia
- Oedema
- Denervation
- Localized destructive disease, e.g. malignant change of TB

IMPORTANT CLINICAL FEATURES OF AN ULCER[12]

- Size, shape, position, edge, base, depth, number, temperature, tenderness, discharge
- State of surrounding tissues, relations, presence of lymphadenopathy, local circulation and inflammation

---

Skin conditions associated with gastrointestinal disease[5]
- Aphthous ulcers – hereditary haemorrhagic telangiectasia
- Benign mucosal pemphigoid – blue rubber-bleb naevi
- Vitiligo – malignant papulosis
- Pyoderma gangrenosum – Henoch–Schönlein purpura
- Dermatitis herpetiformis – Kaposi's sarcoma
- Acrodermatitis enteropathica – pseudoxanthoma elasticum
- Behlet's syndrome – Ehlers–Danlos syndrome

SKIN CONDITIONS WHICH RAISE THE POSSIBILITY OF SYSTEMIC MALIGNANCY[5]

- Acanthosis nigricans – arsenical keratosis/pigmentation/basal cell epithelioma
- Dermatomyositis – reticulohistiocytoma
- Acquired ichthyosis – carcinoid
- Acquired hypertrichosis lanuginosa ('malignant down') – palmoplantar keratoderma (Howell–Evans syndrome)
- Pachydermoperiostosis – Gardner's syndrome
- Exfoliative dermatitis/erythroderma – Peutz–Jeghers' syndrome
- Bowen's disease – thrombophlebitis migrans
- Erythemas (erythema gyratum repens/glucagonoma syndrome) – multiple seborrhoeic keratosis

13

ORTHOPAEDICS

ARTHRITIS

OSTEOARTHRITIS

Commonest causes of secondary osteoarthritis[22.287/8]

- Obesity
- Abnormal contour of the articular surfaces, particularly malunited surfaces
- Malalignment of the joints from deformity, fracture or the distortion of the anatomy by previous surgery, particularly meniscectomy of the knee
- Joint instability due to trauma or generalized ligamentous laxity
- Genetic or developmental abnormalities, such as epiphyseal dysplasia, Perthes' disease or slipped epiphysis
- Metabolic or endocrine disease, including ochronosis (alkaptonuria), acromegaly and the mucopolysaccharidoses
- Inflammatory diseases such as rheumatoid arthritis, gout and infection
- Osteonecrosis
- The neuropathies, especially denervated joints and Charcot's disease

In short, any joint disease can cause osteoarthritis!

Stages in the development of osteoarthritis

- Breakdown of the articular surface
- Synovial irritation
- Remodelling
- Eburnation of bone and cyst formation
- Disorganization

Grading of osteoarthritis

- **I** – superficial damage to the load-bearing cartilage, early fibrillation, pitting, grooving and blisters
- **II** – more extensive destruction of the cartilage with deeper fibrillation and flaking, early osteophytes
- **III** – total loss of cartilage, eburnation, fibrillation, flaking, sclerosis and deformation of the articular surfaces with osteophyte formation
- **IV** – the above, plus osteophytes prominent wit remodelling of the bone ends. Capsular fibrosis leads to fixed deformities

Treatment of osteoarthritis[22.294]

- Drugs and operation are sometimes needed for patients with osteoarthritis, but not always
- Management depends on careful assessment of the precise local and general problems for the patient
- Simple, non-invasive measures are often the best
- Much depends on a positive and optimistic approach
- Polypharmacy and multiple operations should be avoided, but the belief that nothing can be done may be just as damaging

Types of arthroplasty[22]

- Excision
- Interposition
- Mould
- Replacement, including hemiarthroplasty and total replacement

RHEUMATOID ARTHRITIS

Treatment

The aim is to:

- Relieve pain
- Improve function
- Prevent further deterioration

Conservative measures in rheumatoid arthritis[22]

- Drugs
- Rest during an acute attack and mobilization during remission
- Aids and appliances

Indications for operation in rheumatoid arthritis[22]

- To remove inflamed synovium by synovectomy
- To repair damaged soft tissue
- To salvage destroyed joints

Surgical options

- Synovectomy, osteotomy, soft tissue release, tendon repair and transfer, arthroplasty and arthrodesis
- Essential surgery
  - C1–C2 subluxation with neurological signs
  - Compression neuropathy
  - Infected nodules or joints
  - Rupture or threatened rupture of tendon

SEPTIC ARTHRITIS (SEE SURGICAL INFECTION: PAGE 37)

OTHER BONE DISEASE

CAUSES OF BONE NECROSIS[20,22]

- Interruption of arterial supply
  - Fracture (including spontaneous osteonecrosis)
  - Dislocation
  - Infection
- Arteriolar occlusion
  - Sickle cell disease and thalassaemia
  - Vasculitis
  - Caisson disease
- Capillary compression
  - Gaucher's disease
  - Fatty infiltration (due to corticosteroids or alcohol abuse)

MAIN TYPES OF OSTEOCHONDRAL LESIONS[22]

- Osteochondral fractures
- Chondral flaps and separations
- Osteochondritis dissecans
- Spontaneous osteonecrosis
- Osteochondritis dissecans of the lateral condyle

TYPES OF OSTEOCHONDRITIS

- Crushing
  - Metatarsal – Freiberg's
  - Navicular – Kohler
  - Lunate – Kienbock
  - Capitulum – Panner
- Splitting
  - Femoral condyle
  - Elbow capitulum
  - Talus
  - Metatarsal
- Pulling
  - Tibial tuberosity – Osgood-Schlatter
  - Calcaneum – Sever
  - ?Spine – Scheuermann's

CAUSES OF BONE DEFORMITY[20]

- Congenital disorders, e.g. pseudoarthritis
- Bone softening, e.g. rickets, osteomalacia
- Dysplasia, e.g. multiple exostosis
- Growth plate injury
- Fracture malunion
- Paget's disease

CAUSES OF JOINT DEFORMITY[20]

- Contracture of overlying soft tissue
  - Skin, e.g. burn
  - Fascial, e.g. Dupuytren's
  - Muscle, e.g. Volkman's ischaemic necrosis
- Muscle imbalance, e.g. neurological disorder
- Joint instability, e.g. torn ligament, dislocation, chronic arthritis
- Joint destruction, e.g. chronic arthritis

OSTEOPOROSIS

Aetiology[20]

- Primary
  - Post-menopausal
  - Senile

- Secondary
  - Immobilization
  - Nutritional
    - Scurvy
    - Malnutrition
    - Malabsorption
  - Endocrine
    - Hyperparathyroidism
    - Gonadal insufficiency
    - Cushing's disease
    - Thyrotoxicosis
  - Drug-induced
    - Corticosteroids
    - Alcohol
    - Heparin
  - Malignant disease
    - Carcinomatosis
    - Multiple myeloma
    - Leukaemia
  - Non-malignant
    - Rheumatoid arthritis
    - Ankylosing spondylitis
    - Tuberculosis
    - Chronic renal disease
- Idiopathic
  - Juvenile osteoporosis
  - Post-climacteric osteoporosis

Comparison between osteoporosis and osteomalacia[20]

Osteomalacia	Osteoporosis
Both common in ageing women	
Both prone to pathological fracture	
Both decreased bone density	
Ill	Not ill
Generalized chronic ache	Pain only after fracture
Muscles weak	Muscles normal
Looser's zones	No Looser's zones
Alkaline phosphate increased	Normal
Serum phosphate decreased	Normal
Ca × P <2.4mmol/l	Ca × P >2.4 mmol/l

DYSTONIA AND NEUROPATHY

CAUSES OF DYSTONIA[20]

- Generalized
  - Cerebral disorders, e.g. cerebral palsy, stroke and Huntingdon's disease
  - Drug-induced
- Focal
  - Stroke (hemiplegia or monoplegia)
  - Spasmodic torticollis
  - Writer's cramp

CAUSES OF POLYNEUROPATHY[20]

- Hereditary
  - Hereditary motor and sensory neuropathy
  - Friedreich's ataxia
  - Hereditary sensory neuropathy
- Infections
  - Viral
  - Herpes zoster
  - Neuralgic amyotrophy
  - Leprosy
- Inflammatory
  - Acute inflammatory polyneuropathy
  - Guillain–Barr, syndrome
  - Systemic lupus erythematosus
  - Sarcoidosis
- Nutritional and metabolic
  - Vitamin deficiencies
  - Diabetes
  - Myxoedema
  - Amyloidosis
- Neoplastic
  - Primary carcinoma
  - Myeloma
- Toxic
  - Alcohol
  - Lead
- Drugs

PERIPHRAL NERVE ENTRAPMENT SYNDROMES[22]

Nerve and site of compression:

Upper limb

- Cervical spondylosis
- Suprascapular nerve – suprascapula notch
- Thoracic outlet syndrome – cervical rib or a fibrous bands arising from it, post-fixing of the brachial plexus, hypertrophy or spasm of the scalenus anterior

- Median nerve
  - Ligament of Struthers running from 5 cm above the elbow to the medial epicondyle
  - Pronator teres muscle
  - Flexor digitorum sublimis or bands affect the anterior interosseus nerve 5–8 cm below the lateral epicondyle
  - Carpel tunnel
- Ulnar nerve
  - Flexor carpi ulnaris (Cubital tunnel syndrome)
  - Guyon's canal between the hamate and the pisiform
- Radial nerve
  - Rare. Arcade of Frohse affecting the posterior ineroseous nerve and leads to Supinator syndrome
  - Lateral epicondyle insertion (Radial tunnel syndrome)
- Combined lesions

Lower limb

- Lateral femoral cutaneous nerve – inguinal ligament
- Sciatic nerve entrapment – rare. Piriformis (Piriformis syndrome)
- Peronealnerve entrapment – fibular tunnel
- Tarsal tunnel
  - Anterior – superficial fascia of the ankle
  - Posterior fascia around the medial malleolus

INFECTION

OSTEOMYELITIS

Aetiology

- Neonates and children – haematogenous spread from a primary focus elsewhere. *Staphylococcus aureus* is the most common organism, streptococci and Gram-negative organisms are less common. In those with sickle cell disease *Salmonella* and *Escherichia coli* may be causative.
- Adults – secondary to a compound fracture. *Staphylococcus* predominates.

Investigation

- FBC, ESR, MSU, blood cultures, throat swab, anti-staphylococcal and anti-streptococcal titres, CXR, bone radiographs may be normal for up to 14 days after the onset of symptoms
- Isotope bone scan

Treatment

Neonatal

- The patient is often septicaemic and requires large doses of parenteral antibiotics such as erythromycin and fusidic acid
- If there is no marked improvement within 24 h surgical exploration and drainage should be considered to prevent diaphyseal ischaemia

Older children and adults

- There is controversy over early surgery
- Advantages of early surgery
  - Early confirmation of clinical diagnosis
  - Pus is obtained for microbiology
  - Early surgical decompression reduces the risk of ischaemic bone damage
- Disadvantages of early surgery
  - Patient's general condition may be poor
  - Operation is frequently unnecessary for simple subperiosteal infections
- Exploration of the medullary cavity may cause spread of a localized infection
- Suggested treatment depends on the clinical situation:
  - If diagnosis is suspected commence parenteral antibiotics (e.g. erythromycin and fusidic acid)
  - If after 48 h there is no sign of clinical improvement (temperature, P, BP and ESR) perform surgical exploration and decompression
  - Antibiotics, suitable to the sensitivities of the organism isolated, should be continued for 3 months
- Complications
  - Septicaemia can be fatal if untreated
  - Acute suppurative arthritis
  - Chronic osteomyelitis (discharging sinuses, sequestrum formation, bone deformity and pathological fractures, amyloidosis)
- Treatment of chronic osteomyelitis
  - Mainly conservative with antibiotic therapy for acute symptoms
  - Sequestrectomy for a persistently discharging sinus
  - Brodie's abscess should be excised and the cavity curetted
  - Antibiotics can be left *in situ* in various forms (e.g. Gentamicin beads)
- Treatment of osteomyelitis of the vertebral column
  - Infection may be pyogenic (*S. aureus*, *E. coli*, *Klebsiella*, *Proteus* or *Pseudomonas* spp.). *Brucella* should be exclude in high-risk individuals and TB should be considered
  - A needle biopsy may be used to identify the causative organism
  - Treatment initially is mainly conservative with bed rest and large doses of parenteral antibiotics
  - Surgical exploration is used when there has been no satisfactory response to conservative Rx
  - Patients should remain on bed rest for 6 weeks followed by mobilization in a plaster jacket, and antibiotics should be continued for 3 months

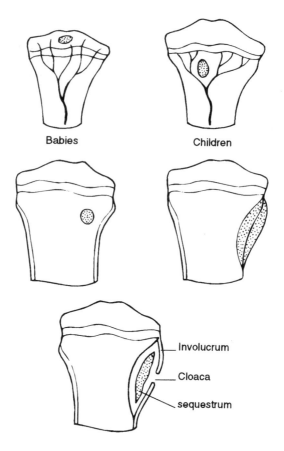

Figure 13.1 Stages in the progression of osteoarthritis. In babies infection may settle near the end of the bone causing joint infection and growth disturbance. In children metaphyseal infection is usual as the growth disk acts as a barrier to the spread of the disease. Infection in the metaphysis may spread to form a subperiosteal abscess. The bone may die and be encased in periosteal new bone as a sequestrum. The encasing involucrum is sometimes perforated by sinuses called cloaca.

SEPTIC ARTHRITIS

Aetiology

- Blood-borne infection from a primary focus elsewhere
- A penetrating injury of a joint cavity
- Secondary to adjacent intraosseous infection
- Organisms
  - *Staphylococcus aureus*
  - *Haemophilus influenzae* (in patients <3 years of age)
  - *Salmonella*
  - Tuberculosis

Clinical features

- Acute, painful, swollen red joint
- Decreased range of movements
- Single joint: hip common in children; knee in adults
- Systemic deterioration (sepsis)

Investigation

- Full blood count, ESR
- Blood cultures
- Joint aspiration and pus culture
- Anti-staphylococcal and anti-streptococcal titres
- Isotope bone scan

Treatment

- Aspiration and irrigation of joint under anaesthesia
- Systemic antibiotics. High-dose parenteral antibiotics (commence with erythromycin and fusidic acid until sensitivities are known). Antibiotics should be continued for 3 months.
- Local splintage

Diagnosis on examination of synovial fluid[20]

Suspected condition	Appearance	Viscosity	Cells	Crystals	Biochemical	Bacteria
Normal	Clear yellow	High	Few	–	As for plasma	–
Septic arthritis	Purulent	Low	White Cells +++	–	Glucose low	+
TB arthritis	Turbid	Low	White cells +	–	Glucose low	+
Rheumatoid arthritis	Cloudy	Low	White cells ++	–	–	–
Gout	Cloudy	Normal	White cells +++	–	Urate	–
Pseudo gout	Cloudy	Normal	White cells +	+	Pyrophosphate	–
Osteoarthritis	Clear yellow	High	Few	+	often	–

MISCELLANEOUS

DIFFERENCES BETWEEN GOUT AND PSEUDOGOUT[20]

Gout

- Smaller joints
- Intense pain
- Inflammation
- Hyperuricaemia
- Uric acid crystals

Pseudogout

- Large joints
- Moderate pain

- Swelling
- Chondrocalcinosis
- Calcium pyrophosphate crystals

TYPES OF REPETITIVE STRAIN INJURY

- Tenosynovitis
- Stenosing tnosynovitis – DeQuervain's affects the long adductor and short extensor of the thumb (Figure 13.2)
- Tendonitis
- Flexor carpi radialis tendinitis
- Carpel Tunnel Syndrome
- Upper limb enthesopathies – golfer's and tennis elbow

REFLEX SYMPATHETIC DYSTROPHY (ALGODYSTROPHY, SUDECK'S ATROPHY)

An exaggerated central and peripheral nervous system response to a painful stimulus usually affecting an extremity.

Characteristics

- Gradual pain
- Swelling

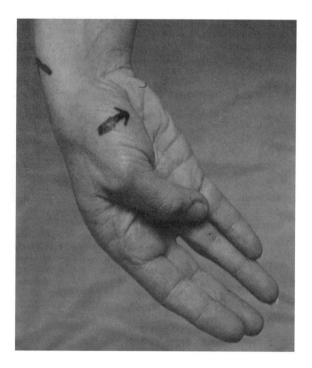

Figure 13.2 Finkelstein's manouevre to diagnose DeQuervain's tenosynovistis. From: *Sports Medicine: Problems and Practical Management* (Eds E. Sherry & D. Bokor); Greenwich Medical Media, 1997: page 177.

- Reduced movement
- Vasomotor skin changes – increased blood flow leads to warmth and erythema with hyperhidrosis after a few months reduced blood flow can occur
- Sensory changes
- Psychological factors – depression or anxiety

Treatment

- Physiotherapy
- Transcutaneous nerve stimulation – 57% of patients find improvement
- Sympathetic blockade
- Psychological support
- Pharmacological, e.g. NSAIDs, corticosteroid and propanolol

SPINE

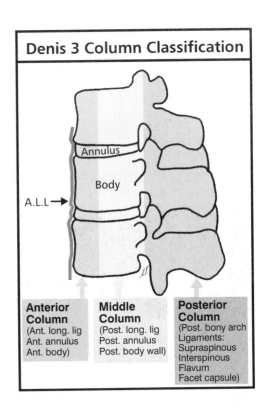

Figure 13.3 Structural elements of the spine. Denis column classification showing the three columns. From: *Sports Medicine: Problems and Practical Management* (Eds E. Sherry & D. Bokor); Greenwich Medical Media, 1997: page 119.

CATEGORIES OF LOW BACK PAIN[9]

- Spondylogenic
- Neurogenic
- Discogenic
- Psychogenic
- Transient
- Visceral

AETIOLOGY OF LOW BACK PAIN[21]

Spinal

- Mechanical
  - Degeneration and displacement (prolapse) of intervertebral disc
  - Spondylosis
  - Spondylolisthesis
  - Scoliosis
  - Instability syndromes
- Tumours – secondary, e.g. breast, bronchus, prostate, thyroid, kidney
- Infection
  - Discitis
  - Osteomyelitis, pyogenic or TB
- Ankylosing spondylitis
- Central spinal stenosis
- Soft tissue ligamentous injuries

Referred

- Infection – urinary, biliary or female genital tract
- Tumours of abdomen or pelvis
- Abdominal aortic abdomen

TYPES OF SCOLIOSIS[22]

- Non-structural (postural) curves due, for example, to limb inequality. There is no rotation of the vertebrae with these curves.

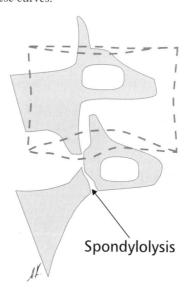

Spondylolysis

Figure 13.5 The 'Scottie dog with collar' found on oblique view in a stress fracture of spondylosis. From: *Sports Medicine: Problems and Practical Management* (Eds E. Sherry & D. Bokor); Greenwich Medical Media, 1997: page 121.

- Structural curves have rotation and sometimes wedging of the vertebrae and they can be divided into:
  - Idiopathic scoliosis
  - Congenital and infantile
  - Neuromuscular
  - Miscellaneous

TYPES OF SPONDYLOLISTHESIS

- **Type I** – Dysplastic. Congenital abnormality of the upper sacrum or arch of L5 allowing slipping (olisthesis) of L5/S1.
- **Type II** – Isthmic. A lesion in the pars articularis usually as a result of a stress fracture or elongation during healing.

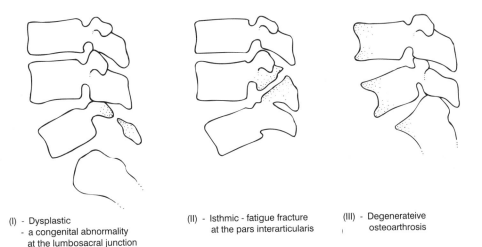

(I) - Dysplastic
    - a congenital abnormality
      at the lumbosacral junction

(II) - Isthmic - fatigue fracture
       at the pars interarticularis

(III) - Degenerateive
        osteoarthrosis

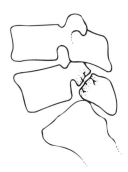

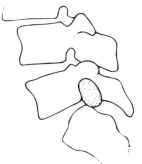

(IV) - Traumatic acute trauma

(V) - Pathological - weakening of the pars
      interarticularis by a tumour, osteoporosis, trauma
      or Paget's Disease

Figure 13.4 Types of spondylolisthesis.

- **Type III** – Degenerative. Can cause unilateral nerve compression or cauda equina compression.
- **Type IV** – Traumatic. Fractures in areas other than the pars.
- **Type V** – Pathological. Generalized or localized bone disease.
- **Type VI** – Post-surgical. Due to loss of bony or discogenic support secondary to surgery

Meyerding classification of slippage grade from I to IV in 25% increments, grade IV being 75–100%.

INDICATIONS FOR SPINAL OPERATIONS[22]

- Disc excision for proven disc protrusions with neurological signs
- Instability caused by spondylolisthesis or unstable discs
- Scoliosis, kyphosis and other spinal deformities
- Tumours and infections

Note: backache is not included.

PROLAPSED INTRAVERTEBRAL DISC

- A tear in the annulus fibrosus allows herniation of the nucleus pulposus. This is usually secondary to a flexion–rotation injury and it commonly affects the L4/5 and L5/S1 disc levels.
- Patients usually present with low back pain, pain in the leg in the L5 or S1 distribution, limitation on straight leg raising and a positive stretch test.
- Signs of L5 root compression:
  - Decreased sensation in L5 dermatome
  - Weakness of extensor hallucis longus, dorsiflexion of ankle and wasting of extensor digitorum brevis
- Signs of S1 root compression:
  - Decreased sensation in the S1 dermatome
  - Weakness of the plantar flexion of the ankle and eversion of the subtalar joint
  - Absent or diminished ankle jerk reflex

DIFFERENTIAL DIAGNOSIS OF PROLAPSED DISCS[22]

- Tumours within the spinal canal
- Neurofibromata in the root canal
- Ependymoma and other tumours
- Intracranal tumour
- Ankylosing spondylitis
- Intrapelvic mass
- Osteoarthritis of the hip
- Spondylosis
- Malingering
- Vertebral tumours
- Tuberculosis
- Infective discitis
- Intermittent claudication

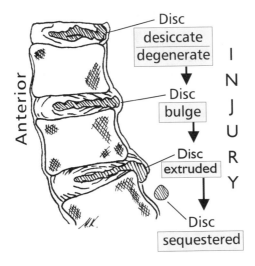

Figure 13.6 Pathophysiology of lumbar disc injury. From: *Sports Medicine: Problems and Practical Management* (Eds E. Sherry & D. Bokor); Greenwich Medical Media, 1997: page 111.

Treatment

- Conservative (most patients symptoms settle with this) – best rest for 2–3 weeks, NSAIDS, analgesics, muscle relaxants, e.g. diazepam, physiotherapy
- Surgical (fenestration, discectomy or microdiscectomy)
  - Indications – failure to respond to conservative Rx, recurrent symptoms ruining life or work, etc., large central disc protrusion causing sphincter disturbance
  - Perform a radiculography, CT or MRI to confirm site of protrusion
  - Chemonucleolysis (using chymopapain in early prolapse). This proteolytic enzyme is injected directly into the disc (anaphylaxis can result)

CAUSE OF SPINAL DYSFUNCTION[2]

- Acute surgery
  - Vertebral fractures
  - Fracture–dislocation
- Infection
  - Epidural abscess
  - Poliomyelitis
- Intervertebral disk prolapse
  - Sequestrated disc
  - Disc prolapse in spinal stenosis
- Vertebral canal stenosis
  - Congenital stenosis
  - Acquire stenosis
- Vertebral bone disease
  - Tuberculous spondylitis
  - Metastatic disease

- Spinal cord tumours
  - Neurofibroma
  - Meningioma
- Intrinsic cord lesions
  - Tabes dorsalis
  - Syringomyelia
  - Other degenerative disorders
- Miscellaneous
  - Spina bifida
  - Vascular lesions
  - Multiple sclerosis
  - Haemorraghic disorders

SHOULDER AND UPPER ARM

CAUSES OF SHOULDER PAIN[20]

- Referred pain syndromes
  - Cervical spondylosis
  - Mediastinal pathology
  - Cardiac ischaemia
- Joint disorders
  - Glenohumeral arthritis
  - Acromioclavicular arthritis
- Bone lesions
  - Infection
  - Tumours
- Calcific tendonitis
- Shoulder impingement syndromes
  - Subacromial (suprasinatus syndrome)
  - Subcoracoid
- Rotator cuff tendonopathies (instability – disloation and subluation)
  - Acute massive rupture with fracture of the greater tuberosity
  - Acute massive rupture without fracture
  - Acute on chronic massive rupture
  - Chronic rupture
- Frozen shoulder – adhesive capsulitis
- Biceps tenosynovitis
- Subacromial bursitis – subacromial 'painful arc syndrome' between 60 and 120° of abduction
- Glenohumeral arthritis
- Acromio clavicular joint disorder 'painful arc' in the last 30° of elevation
- Nerve injury

Anatomical Reconstructions	
Bankart Repair	The anterior detached capsule and labrum reattached.
Capsuloraphy	Stretched or redundant capsule is tightened by placation.
Inferior Capsular Shift	Similar to capsuloraphy but mobilisation of the capsule extends inferiorly to take up redundant inferior pouch. Done in patients with very lax shoulders.
Anatomical Reconstructions	
Putti-Plan	The anterior capsule and subscapularis muscles are divided, overlapped and tightened. Similar to converting a single-breasted coat to a double-breasted coat. This decreases external rotation of the arm
Bristows Procedure	The coracoid process is detached from the scapula and screwed onto the antero-inferior glenoid neck to give extra support to the shoulder
Magnusen-Stack Procedure	The subscapularis, capsule and a portion of the lesser tuberosity is detached and fixed more laterally on the humeral head. This tightens the anterior shoulder structures, decreasing external rotation.

Figure 13.7 Types of shoulder reconstruction.

PAINFUL DISORDERS OF THE ELBOW AND FOREARM

- Tennis elbow – trauma or degeneration at the common extensor muscle origin on the lateral epicondle
- Golfer's elbow – trauma or degeneration of common muscle origins at the medial epicondyle
- Olecranon bursitis
- Pitcher's elbow – valgus strain on the ulnar collateral ligament
- Loose bodies – fragments from osteochrondral fractures or osteochondritis dissecans, which is much rarer at the elbow than the knee
- Infection

Aetiology of Carpel Tunnel Syndrome

- External compression of tunnel walls
  - Trauma (Colles' fracture, vibrating mechanism)
  - Rheumatoid arthritis
  - Subluxation of the wrist
  - Acromegaly
- Compression/swelling within tunnel
  - Fluid retention of pregnancy

- Myxoedema
- Benign tumours
- Chronic proliferative synovitis
- Changes in the median nerve
  - Diabetes mellitus
  - Peripheral neuropathy
  - Hypertrophy of the flexor retinaculum

Diagnosis

- Tinel's sign – tapping over the nerve reproduces the symptoms
- Phalen's sign – flexing the wrist for 1–2 min recreates symptoms
- EMG studies
- Exclude – cervical spondylosis or cervical abnormality (ribs, tumour, cysts) producing a higher nerve lesion

Treatment

- Mild – splintage, corticosteroids, diuretics, restricted activity

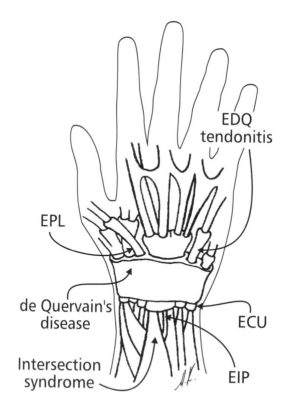

Figure 13.8 Other sites of tendinitis in the wrist and hands. From: *Sports Medicine: Problems and Practical Management* (Eds E. Sherry & D. Bokar); Greenwich Medical Media, 1997: page 177.

- Severe – surgical decompression (note: protect motor branch to thenar muscle by making the incision on the ulnar side of the thenar crease
- Complications – weakness, scar, recurrence, little or no improvement in 10%

HAND INFECTIONS

- Paronychia (nailfold)
- Apical
- Pulp space (felon or whitlow)
- Tendon sheath
    - Signs of Kanavel – flexion
    - Deformity of the digit
    - Uniform swelling and erythema
    - Intense pain on extension and tenderness along the line of the tendon sheath
    - Thenar (thumb) or ulnar bursa (little finger) may become affected
- Web space – infections may force the fingers apart
- Palmar space – deep to the palmar fascia lead to a hand in swollen both aspects and the patient is systemically unwell
- Septic arthritis
- Cellulitis
- Other
    - Orf – sheep workers
    - Erysipeloid – meat workers
    - Pilonidal sinus – hair dressers
    - *Myco. Marinum* – swimming pool attendants

Principles of management of hand infection[9]

- Establish the diagnosis before initiating therapy
- Obtain a culture and give a tetanus booster or vaccination
- Establish adequate anaesthesia; use a tourniquet wherever possible
- Do not inject local anaesthetic into infected tissue
- Incise/excise and drain mature lesions avoiding incisions in 'no-man's land' overlying the distal palm and proximal phalanges
- Elevate the extremity
- Immobilize the extremity with a dorsal plaster splint
- Apply wet dressings to the wound and change frequently
- Use antibiotics in large doses
- Do not close puncture or human bite wounds
- Do not close wounds that have been in contact with dishwater or other contaminated fluids, or in which contamination with sand or dirt has occurred
- Do not drain a felon with a puncture type incision; equally, do not incise every painful digit

Treatment

- Systemic antibiotics
- Drainage of pus (usually at point of maximal tenderness) with irrigation and debridement
- Closed irrigation of tendon sheath infections (two short incisions and placement of a fine catheter for 24 h)
- Elevation and splintage

MANAGEMENT OF ANIMAL BITES

- X-ray to exclude underlying bone injury or foreign body
- Local tissue cleansing – formal exploration and debridement is reserved for extensive, contaminated wounds or where vital structures may be involved
- Delayed primary closure except on the face due to cosmesis and good blood supply
- Tetanus prophylaxis
- Rabies prophylaxis
- Antibiotic prophylaxis is debatable – Co Amoxiclav 500, 125 t.d.s or Doxycycline 200 mg daily in the penicillin allergic (erythromycin for children <12 years of age or breast-feeding mothers) are the drugs of choice

Indications for antibiotic prophylaxis check

Patient indications	Wound indications
Elderly	Crush injury
Splenectimized	<8 h old (delayed primary closure)
Immunocompromized	Bony injury
Immunosuppressed	Puncture wound
Diabetic	Hand/foot injury
	Following primary closure

Human bites

- Management is similar to animal bites except in wounds to the hand and face
- Should be covered by antibiotics (e.g. augmentin). Bites to the metacarpal region should be treated by delayed primary closure after thorough irrigation with iodine

Safe practice in tourniquet application

	Maximum cuff pressure	Maximum ischaemic time
Upper limb	200 mmHg	90 min
Lower limb	300 mmHg	120 min

HIP AND LOWER LIMB

DIAGNOSTIC CALENDAR OF HIP DISORDERS[20,11]

Age at onset (years)	Probable diagnosis
0 (birth)	Congenital dislocation
0–5	Perthes' disease, CDH presenting late, irritable hip, septic arthritis
5–10	Irritable hip, Perthes', infection
10–20	Slipped upper femoral epiphysis, infection
Adult	Osteoarthritis, avascular necrosis, rheumatoid arthritis

CAUSES OF OSTEOARTHRITIS OF THE HIP[20]

- Abnormal stress – defective cartilage; abnormal bone
- Subluxation – infection; fracture
- Coxa magna – rheumatoid; necrosis
- Coxa vara – calcinosis; Paget's
- Minor deformities/protrusion – chondrolysis; other causes of sclerosis

RADIOLOGICAL CHANGES IN OSTEOARTHRITIS OF THE HIP[22]

- Narrowing of the joint space
- Cyst formation in the femoral head and the acetabulum
- Sclerosis of subchondral bone
- Osteophyte formation
- Subcortical thickening on the medial side of the femoral neck
- If there is also bone destruction, Shenton's line will be disturbed, indicating a true shortening of the limb

CONSERVATIVE TREATMENT OF OSTEOARTHRITIS OF THE HIP[22]

- Anti-inflammatory drug
- Weight reduction
- A stick, which is only helpful if it is held in the opposite hand and used correctly
- A raise to the shoe of the shorter limb to correct the apparent shortening and to relieve the abnormal strain on the lumbar spine and the opposite hip
- Aids to daily living to help the patient put on shoes and pick up dropped articles

SUGGESTED GUIDE TO MANAGEMENT OF OSTEONECROSIS OF THE HIP[20]

Stage	Traumatic	Non-traumatic
I	Reduction and fixation	Decompression
II	Bone grafting	Decompression
III	Young osteotomy and grafting	Osteotomy and grafting
	Old joint replacement	Joint replacement
IV	Joint replacement	Joint replacement

KNEE PAIN

Causes

- Patellofemoral overload
- Overuse in athletes
- 'Jump' knee
- Patellofemoral subluxation
- Bipartite patella
- Patella cysts or tumours
- Prepatellar bursitis
- Plica syndrome

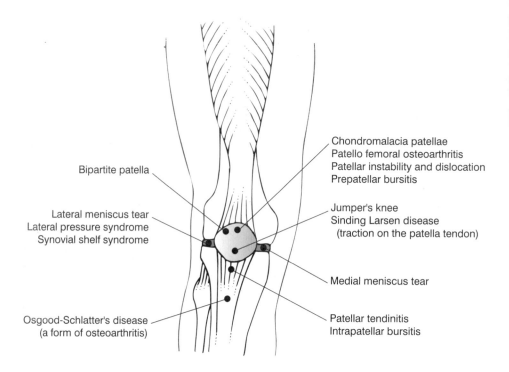

Bipartite patella

Lateral meniscus tear
Lateral pressure syndrome
Synovial shelf syndrome

Osgood-Schlatter's disease
(a form of osteoarthritis)

Chondromalacia patellae
Patello femoral osteoarthritis
Patellar instability and dislocation
Prepatellar bursitis

Jumper's knee
Sinding Larsen disease
(traction on the patella tendon)

Medial meniscus tear

Patellar tendinitis
Intrapatellar bursitis

Figure 13.9 Causes of knee pain.

- Osteochondritis dissecans
- Discoid meniscus
- Torn meniscus

Common internal derangements of the knee[22]

- Meniscus lesions
- Loose bodies
- Chondral separations
- Osteochondritis dissecans

Causes of a 'locked' knee[21]

- Loose intra-articular body
  - Osteophyte formation secondary to osteoarthritis
  - Osteochondral fracture
  - Osteochondritis dissecans
  - Synovial osteochondromatosis
- Meniscal tear

Differences between anterior cruciate rupture and meniscal lesions[22]

- Cruciate symptoms are caused by a high-speed twisting injury with the knee almost straight

- Meniscus lesion by low speed movements with the knee bent
- Ligament injuries usually follow a memorable injury, meniscal injuries seldom do
- Menisci can lock the knee and block extension whereas ligament injuries cause collapse

Signs of a meniscal injury

- Joint effusion
- Tenderness in the joint lie over the affected meniscus
- Positive McMurray's test (a palpable click on rotation at various degrees of flexion)
- Positive Apley compression test (axial loading in the prone patient with the knee flexed at 90°)

Clinical diagnosis of knee instability[31]

Type	Test	Description	Injury to
Straight instability			
	Medial	Abduction laxity tested at 30° of flexion	Medial collateral ligament
	Lateral	Adduction laxity tested at 30° of flexion	Lateral complex tear
	Anterior	Positive anterior drawer sign	Anterior cruciate tear
	Posterior	Positive posterior drawer sign	Posterior cruciate tear
Rotational instability			
	Antero lateral	Positive pivot shift test* Injury to lateral capsular ligament	Anterior cruciate tear
	Antero medial	Positive abduction stress and positive anterior drawer test in external rotation	Anterior cruciate tear Injury to postero medial capsular structures

Pivot shift test – positive if a palpable or visible shift of the tibia is seen between 20° and 30° of flexion as the knee is flexed or extended with the tibia held in external rotation.

Lachman's test – for antecruciate disruption is positive in 85% of cases. Positive if there is an anterior translation of the tibia on the femur at 25° of flexion.

Anterior drawer test – positive if there is abnormal translation of the tibia under the femur with the knee flexed 90°and the foot fixed.

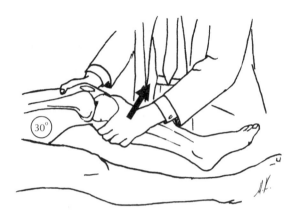

Figure 13.10 Lachman's test is highly specific for anterior cruciate disruption. The knee is flexed to 30° and the upper tibia is moved forward (subluxed) on the lower femur. From: *Sports Medicine: Problems and Practical Management* (Eds E. Sherry & D. Bokor); Greenwich Medical Media, 1997: page 203.

CLASSIFICATION OF FOOT DEFORMITIES[22]

- Forefoot deformities, more common and usually trivial
- Hindfoot deformities, less common and more serious

Hallux rigidus[27]

Treatment

- Conservative
  - NSAIDs and rigid soled footwear
  - Local anaesthetic and corticosteroids followed by manipulation
- Surgical
  - Cheilectomy – excision of the dorsal osteophyte
  - Keller's arthroplasty – 90% success in 5 years
  - Osteostomy – excision of dorsal wedge from the proximal phalanx (Kessel–Bonney operation). Treatment of choice in the young with no osteoarthritis
  - Arthrodesis – 90 % success in 10 years. Toe arthrodesed in 15–20% valgus and 10–15% extension
  - Silicone rubber osteotomy – replacement of base of the proximal phalanx

Hallux valgus[27]

Treatment

- Conservative – larger footwear
- Surgical
  - Bunionectomy – usually combined with a soft tissue procedure
  - Soft tissue procedures – variations on the McBride procedure with release of the adductor hallucis, transverse metatarsal ligament and lateral capsule combined with excision of the medal eminence ad reefing of the capsule
  - Osteotomy – distal: Chevron, Mitchell and Wilson
  - Arthrodesis – cone and socket type with screw fixation

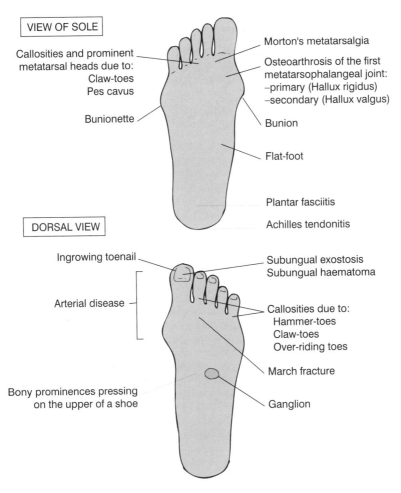

Figure 13.11 Common causes of pain in the adult foot (excluding infections, RA and OA secondary to injury).

- Keller's arthroplasty – excision of the base of the proximal phalanx and trimming of the medial osteophyte

Claw toes[27]

- If it is possible passively to straighten the toes transfer flexor tendons to extensors (Girdlestone's dynamic correction)
- If fixed but not dislocated, divide the metatarsal heads obliquely to make them less prominent (Helal's procedure)
- If fixed and dislocated, perform a forefoot arthroplasty (this will shorten the foot and should be performed bilaterally)

Hammer toes

- Extensor tendons can be divided, the PIP joint excised and stabilized with K wires

CHILDREN

DEVELOPMENT DYSPLASIA OF THE HIP

- Incidence 1:1000 live births. Four times more common in females. Left side is 10 times more frequently involved than the right
- Bilateral DDH is more common than right-sided involvement alone
- Risk factors
  - First born
  - Breech delivery
  - Caesarean section
  - Positive family history
  - Oligohydramnios
- Barlow's test – detects a dislocated hip
- Ortalani's test – detects a dislocated but reducible hip

Radiological investigations of the dysplastic hip

Ultrasound – assesses the acetabulum and position of the femoral head

Radiography is of limited value before ossification of the femoral caital epiphysis at age 4–6 months

- Hilgenreiner's horizontal line – drawn through the triradiate cartilages
- Perkin's vertical line – at right angles to Hilgenreiner's line through the anteriorinferior iliac spines
  - In combination these lines produce quadrants that are used to localize the femoral capital epiphysis
  - Before this ossifies, the metaphyseal beak of the proximal femur will lie in the inner lower quadrant in the normal quadrant
- Acetabular index – angle between Perkin's vertical line and the slope of the acetabular roof. In the newborn it should be $\leqslant 30°$
- Shenton's line – a line following the curve of the inferior margin of the superior margin of the superior ramus down onto the inferior medial border of the femoral neck should be unbroken. Elevation of the lateral part reflects proximal migration of the femoral head and neck
- Teardrop sign (Kohler)
- Femoral capital epiphysis shows delayed appearance and irregular maturation
- Hypoplasia of ipsilateral iliac wing
- Increased femoral neck-shaft angle

Arthrography

- Outlines the articular surfaces, confirms a satisfactory concentric reduction

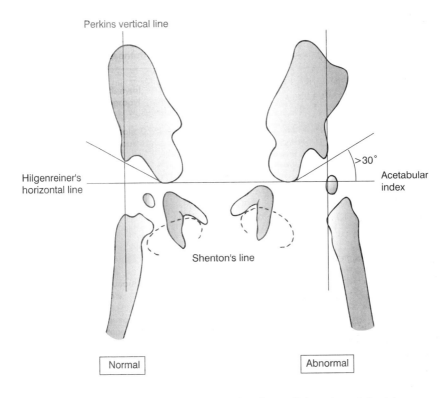

Perkins vertical line

Hilgenreiner's
horizontal line

>30°

Acetabular
index

Shenton's line

Normal

Abnormal

Figure 13.12 Analysis of hip radiographs in dysplastic dislocation of the hip.

TREATMENT OF CONGENITAL DISLOCATION OF THE HIP (CDH, DEVELOPMENT DYSPLASIA OF THE HIP, DDH)11

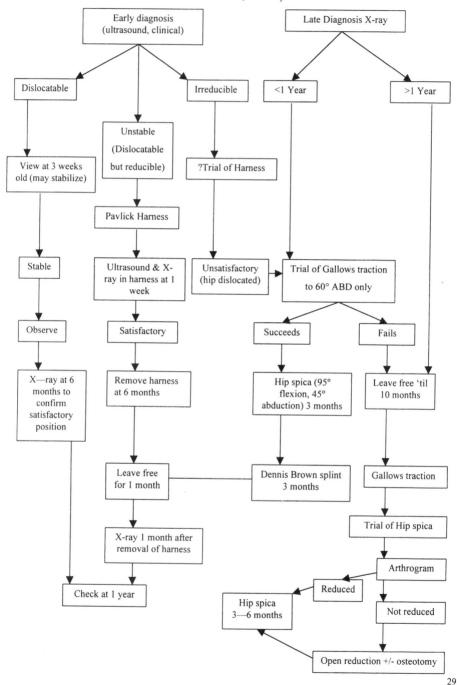

APPROACH TO A LIMPING CHILD[20]

- General assessment – exclude non-accidental injury
- Measure limb length
- Examine the hip for:
  - Septic arthritis, dislocation, subluxation, coxa vara
  - Transient synovitis, Perthes' disease, arthritis, tumour?
- Examine the knee for – swelling: infection, arthritis, tumour, tenderness: injury, infection, instability: patellar subluxation
- Check the foot for – splinter, injury, swollen ankle: infection, arthritis

DIFFERENTIAL DIAGNOSIS OF THE IRRITABLE HIP[20]

- Perthes' disease
- Tuberculous synovitis
- Juvenile chronic arthritis and ankylosing spondylitis
- Slipped epiphysis
- Infective
  - Septic arthritis
  - Osteomyelitis
  - Rheumatic fever

Many children who present with irritable hip have either an infection or synovitis[11].

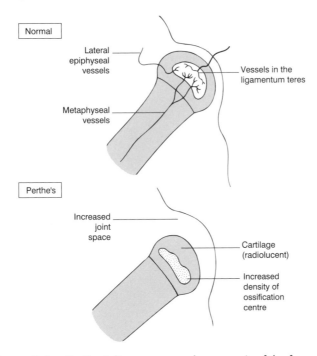

Figure 13.13 Legg–Calve–Perthes' disease: avascular necrosis of the femoral head. The metaphyseal blood supply to the femoral head declines by 4 years of age. Between 4 and 7 years of age the supply may come almost entirely from the layteral epiphyseal vessels. By 7 years of age the vessels in the ligamentum teres have developed.

297

LEGG-CALVE-PERTHES' DISEASE

Results from a gradual compromise to the vascular supply to the femoral head. Incidence is 1 in 10 000. Males are four times more ate risk than females and usually in underprivileged 4–8 year olds with retarded truncal growth.

CLINICAL FEATURES

- Joint irritability
- Pain and limping (intermittent or continuous)
- Abduction (especially in flexion is limited

Diagnosis is apparent from X-ray changes.

TREATMENT OF PERTHES' DISEASE[11]

Treatment is 'containment' of the femoral head in the acetabulum in the hope that it will retain its shape and articular congruence during healing. This is usually achieved by wide abduction in plaster or splints or by a varus osteotomy of the femur or the inominate. Adverse radiological signs are:

- Progressive uncovering of the epiphysis
- Calcification of the cartilage lateral to the ossified epiphysis
- A radiolucent area at the edge of the bony epiphysis (Gage's sign)
- Severe metaphyseal reabsorption

Treatment of Perthes' disease

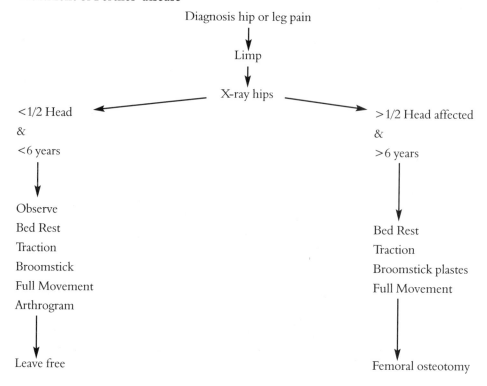

SLIPPED UPPER FEMORAL EPIPHYSIS (SUFE)

The epiphysis of the femoral head can 'slip' off the neck. Incidence is rare (1–3 per 100 000), more common in boys (3:2) and occurs bilaterally in 25% of cases. Peak incidence is related to puberty and occurs about 2 years earlier in girls. Clinical associations occur with hypogonadism (Frohlich's syndrome), hypothyroidism and pituitary dysfunction. Growth hormone is thought to weaken the growth plate and this is therefore weakest at puberty.

Clinical features

- Pain in groin, thigh or knee
- Limp
- 3 types of presentation
  - Commonest – gradual onset over weeks. On examination the child walks with an antalgic Trendelenberg gait with the limb external rotated and shortened. Internal rotation is reduced (particularly in flexion when the limb typically externelly rotates); flexion and abduction are reduced
  - Acute slip – sudden severe symptoms after insignificant traunma
  - Acute on chronic – sudden excacerbation of symptoms on top of a chronic pattern

Investigation

Anteroposterior and true lateral radiographs show:

- a widened and irregular growth plate
- loss of height of the epiphysis
- the 'blanch' sign (a localised increase in density in the metaphysis)

In lateral view:

- the 'Klein' line drawn along the superior cortex of the femoral neck transects less of the epiphysis than the normal side
- if the line passes superior to the head, slippage has occurred (Trethowan's sign)
- the normal right angle between the epiphyseal base and the femoral neck is decreased (anything < 87° is abnormal)
- in a chronic slip, the head slips posteriorly in relation to the neck to produce the appearance of a varus retroverted neck

Aim of treatment

- To preserve blood supply
- To stabilise the physis
- To prevent progressive deformity and accelerated joint degeneration without producing the recognised complications of treatment (e.g. avascular necrosis (AVN) of the femoral capital epiphysis and chondrolysis (hip pain, stiffness, narrowing of joint space)
- To prevent any residual deformity

Treatment

Conservative treatment alone has no role. Active manipulation has a high risk of AVN.

Primary – Fixation of the femoral epiphysis *in situ*, usually with a single screw placed centrally crossing the plate at 90° (Note: severe slips, more than two-thirds the width of the epiphysis on the anteroposterior view or 40° of tilt on the lateral view require specialist treatment as each has a high risk of AVN.)

Secondary – Corrective osteotomy of a deformity if the arc or congruency of the joint are affected.

Salvage treatment – Valgus osteotomy, total joint replacement or athrodesis may be used in severe cases of AVN and chondrolysis.

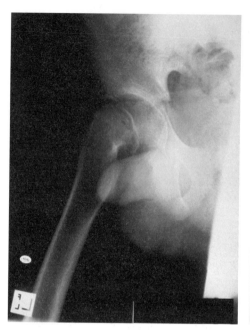

Figure 13.14 Slipped upper femoral epiphysis (SUFE) in an 11 year old.

Figure 13.15 A single screw stabilises the epiphysis and encourages early closure of the growth plate.

From: *Sports Medicine: Problems and Practical Management* (Eds E. Sherry & D. Bokor); Greenwich Medical Media, 1997: page 278.

TREATMENT OF PRINCIPAL DISORDERS OF THE LIMB[20]

	Deformity	Splintage	Surgery
Foot	Equinus	Spring loaded dorsiflexion	Lengthen tendo Achilles
	Equinovarus and dorsiflexion	Bracing in eversion	Lengthen tendo Achilles and transfer lateral half of tibialis anterior to cuboid
Knee	Flexion	Long caliper	Hamstring release
Hip	Adduction	–	Obturator neurotomy
			Adductor muscle release
Shoulder	Adduction		Subscapularis release
Elbow	Flexion	–	Elbow flexor release
Wrist	Flexion	Wrist splint	Lengthen or release wrist flexors

- Genu varum is not physiological if occurring in the over 5's or if the intercondylar distance is >8 cm
- Geno valgum in a child <1 year or with an intermalleolar distance of 10 cm is abnormal

TREATMENT OF 'CLUB FOOT'[11]

- Talipes equinovarus require active treatment and should be distinguished from Talipes calcaneovalgus
- *Conservative* – serial plasters for 6 months or stretching and strapping for 6 months. Night splints after that, if corrected
- *Operative management* – posteromedial release at 9 months for uncorrected club foot, followed by plaster and immobilization and night splints

MANAGEMENT OF LIMB INEQUALITY[22]

- <2 cm at maturity – no treatment
- 2–5 cm – raise to shoe
- >5 cm – operation sometimes

OTHER EXAMPLES OF CONGENITAL DEFORMITY[23]

- Reduction deformities – part or whole of a limb
- Hemimelias – absence of one or other component of a limb, e.g. hypoplasia of radius in Radial club hand
- Fusion of digits – minor or severe, e.g. lobster claw hand
- Trigger thumb – constriction of the tendon sheath opposite the head of the metatarsal (treat by dividing)
- Discoid menscus – treat by excision
- Congenital dislocation, e.g. of the knee (rare)
- Sprengel's shoulder – high scapula and omovertebral bar

NEUROMUSCULAR DISORDERS[27]

Cerebral palsy (see below)

- Incidence 1/1000 live births
- Non-progressive brain disorders causing impairment of motor function

Classification of cerebral palsy

Neurological	Anatomical
Spastic 70%	Hemiplegia 35%
Athetoid 10%	Diplegia 35%
Ataxic	Quadriplegia 30%
Atonic 8%	(Total body involvement)
Rigid	
Mixed7%	

Spina bifida (see below)

Poliomyelitis

- Viral infection affecting the anterior horn cells in the spinal cord and brain stem producing faacd motor paralysis
- Paralysis maximal at 2–3 weeks. Recovery may be complete but any residual paralysis at 6 months is permanent
- Contractures then develop over the next 4–6 months and deformities due to muscle imbalance occur after 1 year

Spinal muscular atrophy

Autosomal recessive. May present at birth or become evident at adolescence Affects anterior horn cells and cranial nerves. Lower limbs are affected more than upper, proximal muscles more than distal.

Hereditary neuropathies

- Peroneal muscle atrophy and Charcot–Marie–Tooth both cause slow progressive distal weakness of the lower limbs.
- Commencing with pes cavus, weakness of the intrinsic muscles of the foot and peroneal muscles leading to a varus deformity and a drop foot with tibialis anterior involvement. Weakness of small muscles of the hand and forearm are late occurrences. If autosomal recessive they occur in childhood if autosomal dominant as adult.
- Freidreich's ataxia is a cerebellar ataxia that has dominant or recessive inheritance causing development of peroneal muscular atrophy, cardiomyopathy, dementia and death.

Arthrogryposis

Characteristized by joint stiffness and contractures to the knee, club foot and hip dislocations probably an intrauterine neuropathy.

Muscular dysrophy

- Duchenne – sex-linked recessive
- Limb girdle dystrophy – autosomal recessive
- Fascioscapulo-humeral dystrophy – autosomal dominant congenital dislocation

SPINA BIFIDA AND MYELOMENIGOCELE[23]

- Failure of the posterior arches to form and close posteriorly
- Often associated with abnormal development of the cord and meninges
- Various degrees exist:
  - *Spina bifida occulta* – common and usually unimportant but can cause cord tethering
  - *Meningocele* – sac continuous with skin may need excision and closure of defect.
  - *Myelomenigocele* – vertebra are defective posteriorly and often malformed resulting in serious spinal deformity (scoliosis and kyphosis). The cord is opened out and functions abnormally (lower limb and truncal paralysis, paralysis of the bladder and anal sphincter). Often associated malformation of the brain stem (hydrocephalus) and other defects (Arnold–Chiari malformation).
- Management (ideally by specialized teams)
  Detailed assessment at birth by orthopaedics, neurologists, paediatricians, social workers, etc. is essential if an accurate prognosis is to be made. Including:

- Accurate assessment of deformities, neurological state of the limbs (motor and sensory)
- Assessment of hydrocephalus
- Assessment of GU tract
- Decide whether the spinal defect should be closed surgically (otherwise death usually results)
- Usually close within 24 h if there is good innervation of the legs as there is a risk of neurological deterioration if closure is delayed
- If hydrocephalus is progressing insert a valve and shunt
- Assess orthopaedic problems
- Deformities may develop due to muscle imbalance (particularly affect the hips and feet). Activities may be restricted by the motor loss
- Joints may lack stability because of muscle weakness
- Limbs may be liable to pressure sores and fractures from lack of normal sensation
- Avoid or correct by splintage or appropriate corrective surgery
- Try to secure muscle balance by partial denervation or tendon transfer
- Use appliances to improve mobility
- Urinary and bowel
  - Control recurrent infections, diversion of ureter, sphincter surgery
  - Concentrate on treatment to those most likely to benefit from it
- Follow up – indefinite

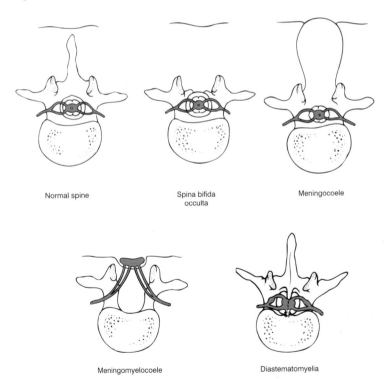

Figure 13.16 Types of spina bifida and dystematomyelia.

CEREBRAL PALSY

- A disorder of movement and posture due to a defect or lesion in the immature brain
- Caused by intrauterine developmental defects, birth trauma and asphyxia, diseases or injuries in early life
- Essentially a motor disorder, but frequently accompanied by other handicaps such as mental defects, blindness, sensory abnormalities and speech defects
- Is a true paralysis as voluntary movements may be weak or absent despite strong muscle contractions
- Usual to find all limbs affected to some extent. Pattern depends on the site. Common types are hemiplegia with joints held flexed and the 'scissoring pattern' with a tendency to extension of joints
- Common disorders are:
  - Spasticity – upper motor neurone type. Reflexes are exaggerated and the stretch reflex is abnormally sensitive. Usually flexors are more spastic than extensors which appear correspondingly weak
  - Loss of coordination
  - Muscle frequently contracts out of phase. Control can be learnt by laborious exercises. Causes difficulties with gait and hand function
  - Athetosis – limbs may move at random with jerking and incoordination
  - Rigidity
  - Hypotonicity – 'floppy infant'
  - Deformity – develops early as a result of muscle imbalance. Common are flexion of the elbow, wrist, fingers and 'clasped thumb', and flexion and adduction deformities of the hip, knee and ankle

Management

- Accurate assessment of problems
- Ideally by specialist teams in specialist centres
- Physiotherapy (e.g. Bobath method)
- Prevent or attempt to correct musculoskeletal deformity
- Train children in posture and movements
- Supervise progress and assist parents

Aim of surgery

- Correct any established deformity
  - Soft tissue division (tendons capsules, skin) and elongation (tendons Achilles', hamstrings, adductors of the hip)
  - Bone correction only when deformities are severe usually simple osteotomies, e.g. through the lower femur to correct a flexion deformity of the knee
- Restore muscle balance and diminish spasticity
  - Tendon lengthening
  - Partial denervation (anterior branch obturator nerve if adductors are over active)
  - Tendon transplantation (usually upper limb)
  - Splintage with callipers
- Surgery is most valuable in the lower limb and may need to be repeated as the child grows
- A child with a normal hand will usually fail to use the other
- Physiotherapy is essential after surgery as even minor procedures may interfere severely with function
- Provide social and psychological support for child and family

JUVENILE CHRONIC ARTHRITIS

- Pauciarticular
  - 70% of presentations. Knee most common, affected joint then ankle. Four times more common in girls
  - Df – involvement of up to four joints within the first 6 months of arthritis
  - High percentage are anti-nuclear antibody-positive
  - 70% will be in remission with little functional disability after 15 years
- Polyarticular
  - 20% of presentation. More common in girls
  - Df – involvement of five or more joints within the first 3 months of onset
  - Tends to persist into adult life and is often classed as juvenile rheumatoid arthritis
- Systemic
  - 10%. Myalgia and arthralgia occurs; arthritis develops later. No sex difference
  - Fever, maculopapular rashes, lymphadenopathy, hetomegay and rarely myocarditis or hepatic dysfunction can develop

Management
- Conservative – physiotherapy, splintage or traction to prevent Contractures. NSAIDs, gold and penecillamine. Intra-articular steroid injections. Cytotoxics in severe cases
- Surgical
  - Soft tissue procedures, e.g. releases of contractures and synovectomy
  - Bony procedures, e.g. epiphyseal stapling for leg length deformity, osteotomies for varus, valgus and flxin deformities or fusions for fixed deformites in older children. Arthrodesis in large joints should be avoided in children with polyarticular disease. Arthroplasty using custom made prothesis is rarely performed in children

BONE TUMOURS

PRIMARY

Classification of primary bone tumours

Tissue	Benign	Malignant
Bone	Osteoid osteoma	Osteosarcoma
Cartilage	Chondroma	Chondrosarcoma
	Chondroblastoma	
	Osteochondroma	
	Osteocartilaginous exostosis	
Fibrous	Aneurysmal bone cyst	Fibrosarcoma
tissue	Fibroma	Malignant fibrous histiocytoma
Marrow	Eosinophilic granuloma	Ewing's sarcoma
		Myeloma
Vascular	Heamangioma	Angiosarcoma
Uncertain	Giant cell tumour	Malignant giant cell tumour
Blood vessels	Haemangioma	Haemangiosarcoma
	Glomus tumour	Haemangiopericytoma
	Angiomatosis	
	Gorham's disease	
Fat	Lipoma	Liposarcoma
		Myxosarcoma
Notochord		Chordoma
Natural	Neurofibroma	Neurofibromasarcoma
elements	Neurofibromatosis	

Clinical features

- Pain
- Hard lump
- Pathological fracture

Investigations

- FBC, ESR, calcium, alkaline phosphatase
- Plain X-rays
- CT or MRI scan
- Biopsy

QUESTIONS TO ASK WHEN LOOKING AT A RADIOGRAPH SUGGESTIVE OF A BONE TUMOUR[20,22]

- Is the lesion solitary of multiple?
- What type of bone is involved?
- Where is the lesion in the bone?
- Is the tumour creating bone or destroying it?
- Is the cortex of the bone intact, broken or eroded?
- If intact, is the cortex thinner than normal and, if so, has it been indented from outside or inside the medullary cavity?
- Are the margins of the lesion well defined? Is there a bony reaction?
- Does the shape of the tumour suggest that it is lifting the periosteum off the bone? If it is, there may be a small triangle of bone at the edge of the tumour, known as *Codman's triangle*, which is often seen in malignant tumours
- Does the lesion contain calcification?

Staging

- **T1** – intracompartmental
- **T2** – extracompartmental
- **G1** – low grade
- **G2** – high grade
- **M0** – no metastases
- **M1** – metastases

- **Stage IA** – T1 G1 M0
- **Stage IB** – T2 G1 M0
- **Stage IIA** – T1 G2 M0
- **Stage IIB** – T2 G2 M0
- **Stage III** – M1, any T, G

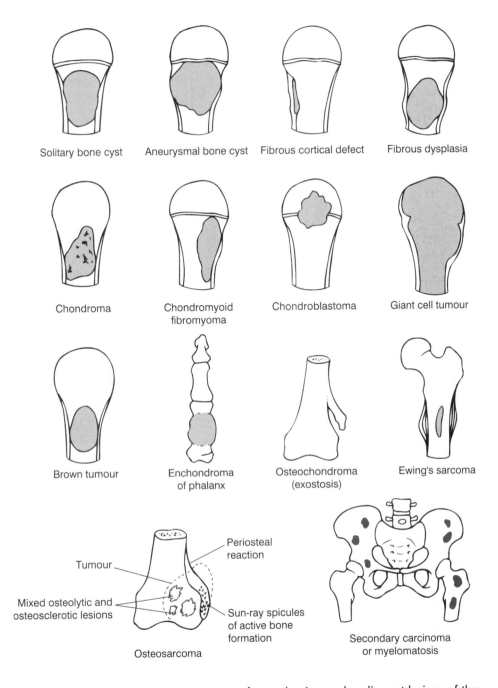

Figure 13.17 Radiographic appearances of cysts, benign and malignant lesions of the bone.

STAGING OF BONE TUMOURS BY ANATOMICAL SITES (T)[9]

Intra-compartmental (T1)	Extra-compartmental (T2)
Intraosseous	Soft tissue extension
Intra-articular	Soft tissue extension
Superficial to deep fascia	Deep fascia extension
Paraosseous	Intraosseous or extrafascial
Intrafascial compartments	Extrafasdcial planes or spaces
Ray of hand or foot	Mid- or hindfoot
Posterior or anterolateral leg	Popliteal fossa
Anterior, medial or posterior thigh	Groin-femoral thigh
Buttocks	Intrapelvic
Volar or dorsal forearm	Mid-hand
Anterior or posterior arm	Antecubital fossa
Periscapular	Axilla
Periclavicular	Paraspinal
Head and neck	

SURGICAL MANAGEMENT

- Local excision or amputation of lesion
- Resection margins determines 'curability'
- Reconstruction surgery/prosthesis

SPECIFIC TUMOURS

Osteoid osteoma
- Unknown aetiology
- Highest incidence in 10–20-year age group
- Radiolucent round or oval focus on X-ray
- Local changes, scoliosis, overgrowth
- Surgical excision of nidus

Chondroma
- Enostotic or exostotic
- Radiologically lucent – sclerotic margins, stippled calcification
- Multiple lesions in syndromes; Olliers', Maffuci

Chondroblastoma
- Adolescent males
- Epiphysis of long bones

Giant cell tumour (osteoclastoma)
- Uncommon
- Multinucleate giant cells histologically
- 20–45 years of age; more common in women
- One-third truly benign, one-third locally invasive, one-third metastasize
- Sites – proximal femur, humerus, fibula, tibia; distal femur, hand
- Radiolucent, with thin cortex

Osteosarcoma
- Peak incidence in 10–25- and 40–50-year age groups
- Second peak related to Paget's disease, radiation therapy
- Sites of rapid growth
  - Distal femoral metaphyses
  - Proximal humerus, tibia, femur
  - Pelvis affected in Paget's disease
- Mixed lytic/blastic X-ray features
  - Elevated periosteum (Codman's triangle)
  - Perpendicular striations(sunburst appearance)
  - 'Onion skin' periosteum
  - Skip lesions within same bone representing tumour spread
  - Incision biopsy (to confirm the diagnosis) then chemotherapy (including high-dose methotrexate)
  - If absence of secondary deposits is then confirmed precede to either:
    - *En bloc* excision and prosthesis replacement (e.g. in long bones), or
    - Limb amputation (long bones) or excision of dispensable bone (scapula or rib)
  - If the tumour has been largely or totally destroyed in the surgical specimen by the preoperative chemotherapy continue the same regime postoperatively – good prognosis (if the tumour cells are still viable switch to second line therapy – poor prognosis)
  - Resection – 15–20% 5YS
  - Resection + chemotherapy – 60% 5YS
  - Worse prognosis with proximal and axial skeleton lesions
  - Adjuvant chemotherapy improves prognosis and allows limb sparing surgery

Chondrosarcoma
- Rare <40 years of age
- Slow progression and late metastasis
- X-ray appearance of irregular calcification in cartilage area

Ewing's tumour
- Rare. Incidence 0.1/100,000
- Arises from vascular endothelium in bone marrow
- Diaphyis of long bone
- Large periosteal reaction
- Peak age 10–20 years of age
- If the primary tumour is excisable in expendable bone, perform a wide excision or resection after a course of combined therapy – 60% 5YS

Multiple myeloma
- Arise from marrow plasma cells
- Usually multiple lesions, occasionally large solitary lesion (plasmacytoma)
- 45–65 years of age
- Constitutional symptoms – cachexia, anaemia, renal damage
- X-ray – multiple lytic lesions
- Raised serum ESR
- Bence–Jones proteins in urine or bone marrow puncture confirms diagnosis
- Treat pathological fractures locally, systemic chemotherapy

Secondary bone tumours

- Primary sites
  - Breast
  - Prostate
  - Lung
  - Thyroid
  - Kidney
  - X-ray – multiple bony lesions, usually lytic except prostate (sclerotic)
  - Indication of advanced disease
  - Palliative care only

SARCOMA

Malignant tumour of soft tissue (extraskeletal connective tissue).

Tissue	Benign	Malignant
Fibrous	Fibroma	Fibrosarcoma
Fibrohistiocytic	Dermatofibroma	Malignant fibrous histiocytoma
Adipose	Lipoma	Liposarcoma
Smooth muscle	Leiomyoma	Leiomyosarcoma
Striated muscle		Rhabdomyosarcoma
Lymph vessels	Lymphangioma	Lymphangiosarcoma
	Cystic hygroma	
Synovium	Giant cell tumour of tendon sheath	Synovial sarcoma
Mesothelial	Localized fibrous mesothelioma	Mesothelioma
Neural	Neurofibroma	Malignant schwannoma
Uncertain	Myxoma	Epitheloid sarcoma

Aetiology

- Overall rare
  - Sporadic
  - Genetic predisposition in certain disorders
    - Von recklinghausen
    - Gardner's
    - Intestinal polyposis
  - Radiation
  - Viral oncogenes – Kaposi sarcoma and AIDS

Clinical features

- Painless lump
- Progressive growth variable speed
- Local invasion
- Lymph node and distant metastasis with increasing grade and size of tumour

Investigations

- Open biopsy to confirm clinical diagnosis
- CT/MRI scan to establish extent and invasion

Staging

G – histological grade
T – tumour size: T1 <5 cm; T2 >5 cm
N – nodes: N0, no positive nodes; N1, positive nodes
M – distant metastasis: M0, no metastasis; M1, metastases present

Stage

IA – G1 T1 N0 M0
IB – G1 T2 N0 M0
IIA – G2 T1 N0 M0
IIB – G2 T2 N0 M0
IIIA – G3 T1 N0 M0
IIIB – G3 T2 N0 M0
IVA – N1 M0
IVB – M1
Stage I – >80% 10YS
Stage IV – <5% 10YS, <10% 5YS

Treatment

- Curative treatment aimed at removal of primary and metastatic disease
- High recurrence rate for wide local excision
- Decreased recurrence for amputation or compartmentectomy
- High morbidity rate
- Most tumours resistant to radiotherapy
- Survival rate may be improved with adjuvant chemotherapy

14

TRAUMA

MODELS OF A&E CARE[14]

Type	Care	Example of injury
Immediate	Initial assessment and resuscitation. Stabilisation prior to transfer	Hypovolaemic shock
Planned	Treatment protocols, agreed with the in-patient team. Subsequent care as in-patient or out-patient	Shoulder dislocation
Shared	Initial care in A&E. Follow up shared with community	Minor burns
Comprehensive	Initial treatment and any necessary follow-up in A&E department	Mallet finger

INITIAL ASSESSMENT AND MANAGEMENT[30]

- Preparation
- Prehospital phase
  - Airway maintenance, control of external bleeding and shock, immobilization of the patient and transport
  - Obtain information needed for triage: time of injury, events relating to and mechanism of injury and patient history
- Inhospital phase (see below)
- Triage

PRIMARY SURVEY

- **A** – airway maintenance with cervical spine control
- **B** – breathing and ventilation
- **C** – circulation with haemorrhage control
- **D** – disability: neurologic evaluation
  - AVPU
    Alert
    Responding to **V**ocal stimuli
    Responding only to – **P**ainful stimuli
    Unresponsive
  - PERLA – **P**upils **E**qually **R**eactive to **L**ight and **A**ccommodation
- **E** – exposure and environmental control: completely undress the patient, but prevent hypothermia

Note: Treatment is rendered on the ABC priority, and life-threatening conditions are identified and management is begun immediately.

RESUSCITATION

- Oxygenation and ventilation
- Shock management

- Management of life-threatening problems identified in the primary survey
- Monitoring
  - Ventilatory rate, pulse oximetry, blood pressure, pulse, electrocardiographic (ECG) monitoring, Glasgow coma scale – baseline investigations
  - FBC, U&E, cross match and arterial blood gases
  - Radiographs of lateral cervical spine, chest and pelvis
- Urinary and gastric catheter (NG tube) placement – urinary catheters are contraindicated in suspected urethral injury (blood at the penile meatus, scrotal haematoma, a high riding prostate). NG tubes should be passed orally or via a correctly positioned nasopharyngeal tube if a cribriform plate fracture is suspected

SECONDARY SURVEY

- Systematic physical examination
  - Head
  - Maxillofacial
  - Cervical spine and neck
  - Chest
  - Abdomen
  - Perineum/rectum/vagina
  - Musculoskeletal
  - Neurological (including a log roll)
- History
  - **A** – **A**llergies
  - **M** – **M**edications currently taken
  - **P** – **P**ast illnesses
  - **L** – **L**ast meal
  - **E** – **E**vents/environment related to the injury
- Mechanisms of injury related to suspected injury patterns
  - Blunt trauma and penetrating trauma
  - Injuries due to burns and cold
  - Hazardous environment
- Appropriate radiographs, laboratory tests and special studies (e.g. peritoneal lavage)
- 'Tubes and fingers in every orifice'
- Re-evaluation
- Records and legal considerations: records, consent for treatment, Forensic evidence
- Definitive care and transfer

AIRWAY AND CERVICAL SPINE

INDICATIONS OF LARYNGEAL FRACTURE

- Hoarseness or voice alteration
- Neck swelling
- Subcutaneous emphysema
- Crepitus at the fracture site
- Haemoptysis

Treatment

- Protect airway
- ?Perform cricothyroidotomy

CERVICAL SPINE FRACTURE

- Consider any cervical injury to be unstable until proved otherwise
- Injuries usually arise where the mobile cervical spine meets the relatively immobile thoracic spine; therefore there is a need to see radiographs of C7/T1
- Real risk of permanent neurological damage (10% of fracture/dislocation of the spine has disc extrusion; therefore perform a full neurological exam, MRI or CT)
- If there is cord compression (i.e. neurology) relieve the compression before applying traction
- A retropharyngeal haematoma >3 mm suggests an underlying fracture

Anatomy of the spine

The spine can be considered to be made up of three columns.(see page 279)

The anterior column consists of:

- Vertebral bodies, the intervertebral discs and the longitudinal ligament (anterior spinal ligament)

The intermediate column consists of:

- Pars interarticularis, the intervertebral facet joints and ligaments

The posterior column consists of:

- Spinous processes and interspinous ligaments

C1 – THE ATLAS

Jefferson's fracture of the C1 rings from axial compression (i.e. diving) are unstable if they have a lateral spread > 7 mm (open mouth view) as rupture of the transverse ligament has occurred.

Treatment

- Stable – SOMI brace
- Unstable – Halo brace for 3 months
- Occital cervical fusion for persistent instability

C2 – THE AXIS
Odontoid peg fracture

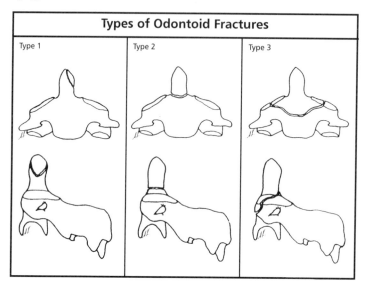

Figure 14.2 Classification of odontoid peg fractures. From: *Sports Medicine: Problems and Practical Management* (Eds E. Sherry & D. Bokor); Greenwich Medical Media, 1997: page 117.

Odontoid peg fracture	Treatment
I – Tip of peg	Stable – soft collar / no treatment
II – Junction with body	Unstable – halo brace or internal fixation
III – Body	Generally stable – SOMI brace

Note: Hangman's fracture (traumatic spondylolisthesis) from hyperextension causing fracture through the pedicles of C2 requires a Halo vest until united (10 weeks).

TYPES OF CERVICAL FRACTURES

- *Anterior fractures* – wedge or burst in type, disrupt the anterior spinal ligament and are relatively unstable
- *Middle fractures* – causing unifacet, bifacet dislocation or fracture dislocation are unstable
- *Post fractures* – fracture the spine or disrupt interspinous ligaments

Note: if only one column is damaged the spine is usually still relatively stable (e.g. wedge, compression fractures). If, however, two columns are involved, an unstable burst or fracture dislocation usually occurs (see page 279 for Denis 3-column classification of the spine).

Radiological classification of cervical spine injury
- Hyperflexion
  - Anterior subluxation

- Bilateral locked facet joints
- Flexion teardrop fracture
- Spinous process fracture (Clay shoveller's fracture)
- Hyperextension
  - Hyperextension strain
  - Fracture of the anterior arch of C1
  - Fracture of posterior arch of C1
  - Hangman's fracture
  - Anterio-inferior vertebral chip fracture
  - Chip fracture
  - Extension tear drop fracture
  - Laminar fracture
- Axial compression
  - Burst fracture
  - Fracture of the pedicles of C2 (Jefferson fracture)
- Flexion rotation injury – unilateral facet dislocation
- Extension rotation injury – pillar fracture

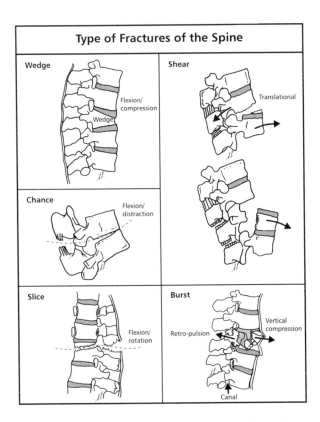

Figure 14.3 Types of fracture of the spine. From: *Sports Medicine: Problems and Practical Management* (Eds E. Sherry & D. Bokor); Greenwich Medical Media, 1997: page 120.

SIGNS OF CERVICAL SPINE INSTABILITY

Consider the fracture unstable if there is:

- Compression of vertebral body >25%
- Kyphotic angulation of >11%
- Loss of vertebral height >25%
- Facet joint widening
- Tear drop fracture
- A base of odontoid peg fracture
- >3 mm space between the front of the odontoid and the back of the anterior arch of the atlas
- Lateral displacement of C1 on C2 >7 mm
- Atlanto occipital dislocation

Treatment

- Protect from secondary injury
- If progressive neurology exists use spinal decompression, then column stabilization
- Unstable in an acceptable position – skull traction (2.5 cm above ear), Halo vest, Minerva jacket (i.e. two columns fractured) or SOMI brace (sterno occipital mandibular immobilizer, cervicothoracic brace)
- Unstable, facet dislocation – traction
- Unstable with unilateral dislocation – fuse
- Protect again secondary problems, i.e. bladder (UTI, renal failure), bed sores, contractures and consider transfer to specialized units

CERVICAL TRACTION

- Using bone callipers, Blackburn callipers, Crutchfield traction tongs
- Weight needed for spinal fracture traction equals sum of level plus one above (lb), e.g. for a C5 lesion C5 +C6 = 11 lb
- Weight needed to reduce dislocation equals five times the level of the vertebra above, e.g. if C4, C5 dislocation 5 × C4 = 20 lb to reduce initially, then 9 lb to provide traction

SPINAL SHOCK

- Produces flaccid paralysis below level of injury. If no return of any function occurs after 48-h prognosis is poor

Classification of cord injury

- Complete, incomplete, none

Partial injuries of the spine

- Cord compression
- Anterior cord syndrome – spastic paralysis, paraparesis (motor loss, sensory intact)
- Posterior cord syndrome – some motor function and crude sensation (motor intact, sensory loss)
- Central cord syndrome – incomplete tetrapareseis (upper limbs more affected than lower). Usually extension injury with no fracture or vascular

- Brown Sequard syndrome – hemisection of the cord ipsilateral paralysis and sensory loss below lesion contralateral analgesia and thermoanaesthesia for a few segments below injury site
- Cord injury without radiological abnormality (concussion, contusion, transection, ischaemia)
- Nerve root compression
- Instability
- Soft tissue injury

Signs that suggest a cervical spine injury

- In the unconscious patient there is:
  - Flaccid areflexia especially with flaccid rectal sphincter
  - Diaphragmatic breathing
  - Hypotension with bradycardia especially without hyovolaemia
  - Priapism an uncommon but characteristic sign
- In the conscious patient there is all of the above, plus:
  - Ability to flex but not extend at the elbow
  - Grimaces to pain above but not below the clavicle

BREATHING

CHEST TRAUMA AND TREATMENT

Injury	Treatment
Uncomplicated rib fracture	Pain relief by non-steroidals, local infiltration or thoracic epidural
Simple pneumothorax	Needle thoracocentesis or chest drainage if severe
Open pneumothorax	Cover wound with an occulsive flutter valve dressing and close surgical
Tension pneumothorax	Needle thoracocentesis and chest drainage
Flail segment	Adequate analgesia, O_2 therapy and i.v. fluids
Haemothorax	Resuscitation and chest drainage blood loss of >200–300 ml/h necessitates thoracotomy. Termed massive if >1500 ml blood is in the thoracic cavity.
Pulmonary contusion	Can lead to ARDS and ventilation
Tracheobroncha tree injuries	Prompt surgical exploration
Cardiac tamponade	Pericardiocentesis, open pericardiotomy
Aortic rupture	Immediate repair
Myocardal contusion	Continuous cardiac monitor, sudden dysrythmias may occur: sinus tachycardia, ventricular ectopics, ST segment changes and right bundle branch block
Oesophageal injury	Chest tube drainage antibiotics and urgent surgical repair
Diaphragmatic rupture	90% is on the left and should be repaired

CAUSES OF POST-TRAUMATIC RESPIRATORY FAILURE[5]

- Obstructive causes
  - Craniofacial injuries
  - Closed head injury – inability to protect airway

- Aspiration/foreign body
- Expanding neck haematoma
- Burns
- Causes of ventilatory failure
  - CNS injury
  - Cord trauma
  - Diaphragmatic rupture
  - Severe flail chest
  - Malnutrition
- Causes of gas-exchange derangements (ARDS)
  - Neurogenic
  - Sepsis
  - Fat embolus
  - Microemboli/shock/massive transfusion
  - Pulmonary contusions
  - Aspiration
  - Inhalation injury
- Oxygen toxicity

CIRCULATION

CHARACTERISTICS OF SHOCK[14]

	HR	BP	CO	Extremities	CVP
Hypovolaemic	↓	↓	↓	Cold	↓
Cardiogenic cold	↑	↓	↓	Cold	↑
Anaphylactic	↑	↓	↓	Rash, sometimes warm at first	↓
Septic	↑	↓	at first, ↓ later	Warm at first, cold later	↓

CLASSIFICATION OF HYPOVOLAEMIC SHOCK ACCORDING TO BLOOD LOSS (BASKETT 1991)[14]

Class	I	II	III	IV
Blood loss (l)	0.75	0.8–1.5	1.5–2.0	2.0
Blood loss (%)	<15%	15–30%	30–40%	40%
Systolic BP	Normal	Normal	Reduced	Very low
Diastolic BP	Normal	Raised	Reduced	Very low
Pulse rate (beats/min)	<100	100–120	120 (weak)	120 (very weak)
Capillary refill	Normal	>2 s	>2 s	Undetectable
Respiratory rate (breaths/min)	Normal	Normal	>20	>20
Urinary flow rate (ml/h)	>30	20–30	10–20	<10
Skin colour	Normal	Pale	Pale	Pale/cold
Mental state	Alert	Anxious, aggressive	Drowsy, aggressive	Drowsy, unconscious

DISABILITY AND SECONDARY SURVEY

TYPES OF HEAD INJURIES

- Primary injury (unable to improve by treatment)
  - Cortical contusions/lacerations
  - Diffuse white matter (axonal) lesions
- Secondary injury (preventable or treatable)
  - Hypoxia
  - Hypovolaemia
  - Cerebral oedema
  - Infection

GUIDELINES FOR THE MANAGEMENT OF PATIENTS WITH HEAD INJURY[14]

Criteria for skull X-ray after recent head injury

The presence of one or more of the following indicates the need for a skull X-ray in patients with a recent history of head injury:

- Loss of consciousness or amnesia at any time
- Neurological symptoms or signs
- Cerebrospinal fluid or blood from nose or ear
- Suspected penetrating injury or scalp laceration, bruising or swelling
- Alcohol intoxication
- Difficulty in assessing the patient (e.g. the young, epilepsy)

Criteria for hospital admission after recent head injury

The presence of one or more of the following indicates the criteria for hospital admission after recent head injury:

- Confusion or any other depression of the level of consciousness at the time of examination
- Skull fracture
- Neurological signs or significant headache or persistent vomiting
- Difficulty in assessing the patient (e.g. alcohol intoxication, the young, epilepsy)
- Other medical conditions (e.g. haemophilia)
- The patient's social conditions or lack of responsible adult/relative

Note: post-traumatic amnesia with full recovery is not an indication for admission. Patients sent home should be given written instructions about possible complications and appropriate action

Criteria for consultation with a neurosurgical unit

The presence of one or more of the following indicates the criteria for consultation with a neurosurgical unit:

- Deterioration
- Depression of the level of consciousness or local neurological signs or fits with or without skull fracture
- Disorientation or other neurological disturbance persisting for >12 h even if there is no skull fracture
- Coma continuing after resuscitation
- Suspected open injury of the vault or the base of the skull
- Depressed fracture of the skull

PREDICTIVE SIGNS OF OUTCOME IN HEAD INJURY PATIENTS[9]

- Favourable signs of recovery in first 72 h
  - Early wakening
  - Verbal response
- Intact caloric response
- Fending off external stimuli
- Normal muscle tone
- Unfavourable signs in the first 72 h
  - Absent spontaneous eye opening
  - Absent spontaneous eye movement
  - Absent pupillary response
  - Absent corneal reflex
  - Absent caloric response
  - Absent deep tendon reflexes
  - Absent muscle tone

Relative risk of intracranial lesion

Low risk	Moderate risk	High risk
Asymptomatic	Change of consciousness	Depressed
Headache	Progressive headache	Consciousness
Dizziness	Alcohol/drug intoxication	Focal signs
Scalp haematoma	Unreliable history	Decreasing
Scalp laceration	Age >2 years	Consciousness
Scalp contusion	Seizure	Penetrating injury
Scalp abrasion	Vomiting	Depressed fracture
Absence of moderate	Amnesia	
or high-risk criteria	Multiple trauma	Serious facial injury
		Signs of basilar injury
		Possible depressed fracture
		Suspected child abuse

RISK OF INTRACRANIAL HAEMORRHAGE[31]

- Orientated with no skull fracture – 1 in 6000
- Disorientated with no skull fracture – 1 in 120
- Orientated with skull fracture – 1 in 32
- Disorientated with skull fracture – 1 in 4

Treatment of traumatic intracranial bleeding

- Extradural (classically with a lucid period after a minor injury followed by a decreasing level of consciousness) – mannitol and frusemide as a holding measure then surgical
- Subdural – surgical
- Intracerebral – conservative management unless deterioration suggests the need for surgical evacuation of the haemorrhage

GLASGOW COMA SCORE

The Glasgow Coma Score forms part of the secondary survey and its true value lies in the observation of trends over time rather than any one value. The adult GCS is well validated but the children's version is not.

Glasgow Coma Score

Eye response (range 1–4)		Verbal response (range 1–5)		Motor response (range 1–6)	
Open spontaneously	4	Orientated	5	Obey commands	6
To speech	3	Confused	4	To pain: localises	5
To pain	2	Inappropriate	3	Normal flexion	4
None	1	Incomprehensible	2	Abnormal flexion	3
		None	1	Abnormal Extension	2
				None	1

Children's Coma Score

For use in children <4 years of age

Eye response	Verbal response (range 1–5)				Motor response	
(as GCS table above)	Smiles, oriented to sounds, follow objects, interacts			5	(as GCS table above)	
	If crying		If interacts			
	Consolable	4	Inappropriately Moaning	4		
	Inconsistently consolable	3		3		
	Inconsolable	2	Irritable	2		
	No response	1	No response	1		

ABDOMINAL INJURY

Aetiology of abdominal injuries[5]

Penetrating	Blunt	Iatrogenic
Stab wounds	Crush injury	Endoscopic
Gunshot wounds	Blast injury	External cardiac massage
Shotgun wound	Seatbelt syndrome	Peritoneal dialysis
		Paracentesis
		Percutaneous transhepatic cannulation
		Liver biopsy
		Barium enema

FREQUENCY OF VISERA AND ORGAN INJURY IN ABDOMINAL TRAUMA[5]

Viscera or organ	In blunt trauma (%)		In penetrating trauma (%)
Spleen	25		7
Kidney	12		5
Intestine	15	Small bowel	26
		Stomach	19
		Colon	17
Liver	15		37
Retroperitoneal (haematoma)	13		10
Urinary bladder	6		
Mesentery	5	(and omentum)	10
Pancreas	3		4
Diaphragm	2		5
Urethra	2		–
Vascular	2		13
Duodenum	–		2
Biliary	–		1
Other	–		1

Diagnosis

- Hx and examination – mechanism of injury, type of trauma, location, of pain and tenderness, PR and PV
- Investigations – FBC, U&E, amylase, X match, pregnancy test
- Plain CXR, AXR – free air in the abdomen or retroperitoneal necessitates a laparotomy
  - Diagnostic peritoneal lavage (see below)
  - Ultrasound – splenic, hepatic and renal injury or to identify free fluid
- Contrast studies depending on injury – ureythrography, cystography, upper or lower GI series, IVU, CT

Diagnostic peritoneal lavage (DPL)

- Indications
  - Equivocal clinical examination
  - Unreliable clinical abdominal examination due to:
    - Reduced consciousness level
    - Influence of alcohol or drugs
    - Neurological impairment, e.g. cervical cord lesion

Accuracy of DPL

- Sensitivity 98% for intraperitoneal bleed
- False-negative rate 2% of cases due to injuries of retroperitoneal, pelvic structures or to ruptured diaphragm
- False-positive rate 2% due to bleeding from pelvic fracture, from operative site or injury to intraperitoneal structures during the procedure

Indicators of a positive DPL

- Red cell count >100,000/mm^3
- White cell count >500 mm^3
- Presence of bile, bacteria, faecal matter

Indications for immediate laparotomy/celiotomy[30]

- Hypotension with evidence of abdominal injury
- Gunshot, stab wounds, blunt trauma with gross blood on DPL
- Peritonitis early or subsequent
- Recurrent hypotension despite adequate resuscitation
- Extraluminal air
- Injured diaphragm
- Intraperitoneal perforation of the urinary bladder on cystography
- Evidence of injury to the pancreas, gastrointestinal tract and injuries to the liver, spleen and/or kidney
- Positive contrast studies of upper and lower gastrointestinal tracts
- Persistent amylase elevation with abdominal findings

Relative contraindications to DPL

- Previous abdominal surgery
- Gross obesity
- Clotting disorders
- Cirrhosis
- Pregnancy

Absolute contraindications

- If a laparotomy is needed

VASCULAR TRAUMA

Types of vascular trauma[30]

- Contusion
- Puncture
- Laceration
- Partial division
- Transection

Indications for surgical exploration of suspected vascular trauma

- Unequivocally
  - Brisk, external bleeding
  - Expanding haematoma (rapid progressive swelling)
  - Abnormal pulses
- Suggestive
  - Bruit or thrill
  - Pallor
  - Empty veins
  - Decreased capillary refill
  - Relative coolness

- Wounds close to the course of a major artery
- Decreased sensation
- Motor weakness
- Progressively increasing pain after immobilization of an extremity injury)

Techniques for repair of vascular injury

- Simple suture – for small holes
- Transverse suture – for small tears
- Patch repair – if stenosis is likely (e.g. internal iliac artery can be used for aortic tears)
- End-to-end anastomosis – for complete transection or a short segment has been damaged
- Interpositional – for significant loss of vessel length

Note: obtain control proximal and distal to injury and perform careful embolectomy before repair is complete.

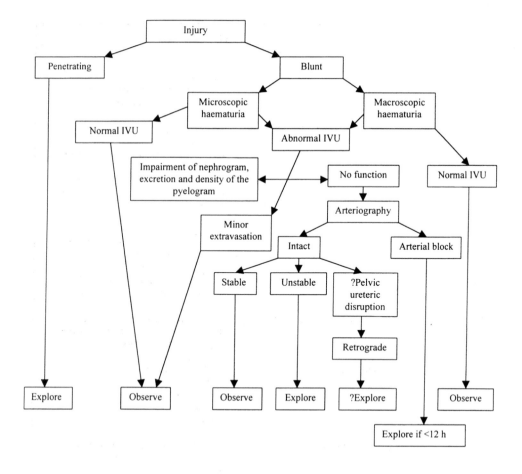

Figure 14.4 Flow diagram showing investigation and treatment of renal injury[5].

METHODS OF REPAIRING A DAMAGED URETER[8]

- If there is no loss of length – spatulation and end to end anastomosis without tension
- If there is little loss of length
  - Mobilize kidney
  - Psoas hitch of bladder
  - Boari's operation
- If there is marked loss of length
  - Transureteroureterostomy
  - Interposition of isolated bowel loop or mobilized appendix
  - Nephrectomy/transplant

SYNOPSIS OF CAUSES OF COLLAPSE TO BE CONSIDERED DURING SECONDARY SURVEY[14]

System	Diagnosis	Notes
Respiratory	Upper airway obstruction	Inhaled foreign body (try Heimlich manoeuvre) Infection such as epiglottitis (occurs in adults although more common in children)
	Trauma including respiratory burns	Call help urgently
	Ventilatory failure	Asthma Chest trauma such as sucking open wound Paralysis such as in Guillain–Barr, syndrome
	Failure of alveolar gas exchange	Pneumonia Pulmonary contusions Cariogenic pulmonary oedema Adult respiratory distress syndrome
	Tension pneumothorax	From trauma (including iatrogenic) ruptured emphysematous bulla
Cardiac	Ventricular fibrillation	Follow Resuscitation Council (UK)
	Asystole	guidelines for treatment of cardiac arrest
	Electromechanical dissociation	Look for treatable cause: tension pneumothorax, cardiac tamponade, hypoxia or hypovolaemia, drug overdose
	Cardiogenic shock or failure	Acute myocardial infarct Arrhythmia Pulmonary embolism Cardiac contusions after blunt chest trauma Valve rupture
Vascular	Hypovolaemic shock	Revealed or concealed haemorrhage Diarrhoea and vomiting Fistulae Heat exhaustion

System	Diagnosis	Notes
	Anaphylactic shock	From stings and bites, drugs or iodine-containing contrast used for radiological investigation
	Dissecting thoracic aorta	Usually in previous hypertensive patients, pain radiates to back
	Leaking abdominal aortic aneurysm	Always check femoral pulse so that you consider aortic pathology (although pulses may not be lost)
	Septic shock	Initially massive peripheral vasodilation: 'warm shock' Temperature may be normal
	Neurogenic shock	From loss of sympathetic vascular tone in cervical or high thoracic spinal cord injury
Gastrointestinal	Haemorrhage	Always check serum amylase
	Perforated peptic ulcer	
	Pancreatitis	Always check serum amylase
	Mesenteric embolism	Abdominal signs may be absent initially
Gynaecological	Ruptured ectopic pregnancy	Usually at 4–6 weeks of gestation Always think of diagnosis in the collapsed young woman
Obstetric	Supine hypotension	Gravid uterus obstructs venous return from the vena cava unless the pregnant woman is turned on her left side
	Eclampsia	
	Pulmonary embolism	
	Amniotic fluid embolism	
Neurological	Head injury	Isolated head injuries do not cause shock in adults. Look for sites of loss of blood elsewhere
	Infection	Meningitis in children (often meningococcal in UK) Tetanus, botulism, poliomyelitis, rabies
-	Cerebrovascular	Intracranial embolism or haemorrhage Subarachnoid haemorrhage may present solely as a severe headache
-	Epilepsy	Including the postictal state
	Poisoning	*Refer to following table*
Haematological	Sickle cell crisis	May lead to respiratory failure
	Malaria	Cerebral malaria causes coma
	Coagulopathy	Thrombocytopenia may present with bleeding
Metabolic	Hypoglycaemia	Check blood glucose in every patient
	Hyperglycaemia	Coma may be first presentation of diabetes mellitus
	Hyponatraemia	May be Addisonian crisis
	Hypocalcaemia	May present with fits

System	Diagnosis	Notes
	Hepatic failure	Precipitated by paracetamol overdose in previously fit people, and by intestinal haemorrhage, drugs, or high-protein diet in those with chronic liver disease
-	Renal failure	Prerenal from dehydration
		Renal, e.g. from crush syndrome and myoglobinuria
-		Post-renal from ureteric obstruction (dangerous hyperkalaemia causes tall tented T waves and widening of the QRS complexes)
	Hypothermia	Resuscitation must include passive or active core rewarming
		Sepsis and hypovolaemia often coexist
Endocrine	Addisonian crisis	Give 200 mg hydrocortisone i.v. (hypotension, low serum sodium, raised serum potassium)
	Myxoedema	Always consider in hyperthermia patients

COMMON DRUGS AND POISONS[14]

Drug	Symptoms and signs	Treatment
Paracetamol	Liver and renal failure, hyperglycaemia	Lavage charcoal or methionine
	May be asymptomatic initially	Acetylcysteine
Salicylates	Tinnitus, abdominal pain	Lavage and charcoal
	Vomiting, hypoglycaemia, hyperthermia, sweating	Rehydration
	Acid-base disturbance	Diuresis
Tricyclic antidepressants	Arrythmias and hypotension	Lavage and charcoal
	Dilated pupils, convulsions	Cardiopulmonary support
	Coma	
Benzodiazepines	Respiratory depression	Flumenazil if acute iatrogenic
Opiates	Pinpoint pupils	Naloxone
	Loss of consciousness	
	Respiratory depression	
	Needle marks	
Phenothiazines	Dyskinesia, torticollis	Procyclidine
Lignocaine	Tingling tongue	Cardiopulmonary support
	Perioral paraesthesia	Diazepam
	Ventricular fibrillation	
	Convulsions	
Carbon monoxide	33% of fatal pisonings in the UK – insidious from inefficient gas fires	
	Nausea and vomiting	

Drug	Symptoms and signs	Treatment
	Headache and drowsiness	
	Hallucinations, convulsions	100% or hyperbaric oxygen
Cyanide	Headache, vomiting, weakness	Dicobalt edetate
	Tachypnoea, convulsions	
	Coma	
Iron	Hypotension, vasodilation	Lavage
	Gastric haemorrhage	Desferroxamine
Organophosphates	Nausea, vomiting, diarrhoea	Lavage
(pesticides, nerve	Salivation, pulmonary oedema	Atropine
gases)	Pinpoint pupils, convulsions, coma	

TETANUS PROPHYLAXIS[14]

Categories of immune status	Action for superficial clean, non-penetrating wounds <6 h old	Action for other wounds
	Surgical toilet for all wounds ↓	Surgical toilet for all wounds ↓
Previous complete course of toxoid or a booster dose within past 5 years	No further treatment	No further treatment
Previous complete course of toxoid or a booster dose between 5 and 10 years ago	One dose toxoid	One dose toxoid
Previous complete course of toxoid or a booster dose 10 years ago	One dose toxoid	One dose toxoid and human tetanus immunoglobulin
No complete course of toxoid or immune status unknown	Complete course toxoid	Complete course toxoid and human tetanus immunoglobulin

TRIAGE, INJURY AND TRAUMA SCORING

Triage prioritises patients before treatment begins. In casualty the number of patients and the severity of injuries should not exceed the available medical resources, so triage selects the more severely injured patient for priority treatment. In large-scale emergencies the number of patients and the severity of injuries could exceed the available medical resources. Triage then identifies those who will be given the best chance of survival with the available resources and time scale

COMMONLY USED TRIAGE CATEGORIES[27]

Colour	P	T	Description
Red	P1	T1	Immediate
Yellow	P2	T2	Urgent – require Treatment within 4–6 h
Green	P3	T3	Delayed – do not require treatment within 6 h
Blue	–	T4	Expectant – patients who are not expected to survive
White	Dead	Dead	Dead

BRITISH NATIONAL TRIAGE SCALE (COMMONLY USED IN A&E DEPARTMENTS)[27]

Colour	Priority	Category	Target time
Red	1	Immediate resuscitation	98% seen on arrival
Blue	2	Very urgent	95% seen within 10 min
Brown	3	Urgent	90% seen within 60 min
Yellow	4	Standard	Within 120 min
Green	5	Non urgent	Within 240 min

TRIAGE SIEVE (USUALLY FOR MASS CASUALTIES)[27]

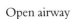

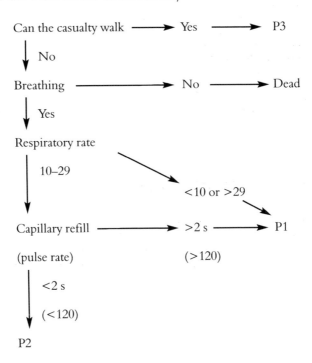

TRIAGE SORT OR TRIAGE REVISED TRAUMA SCORE (TRTS) IS BASED ON THE THREE PARAMETERS OF THE REVISED TRAUMA SCORE (RTS)

- Respiratory rate
  >29 4
  10–29 3
  6–9   2
  1–5   1
  0   0
- Systolic BP
  >90   4
  76–89 3
  50–75 2
  1–49 1
  0   0
- Glasgow Coma Scale
  13–15 4
  9–12 3
  6–8   2
  4–5   1
  3   0

Then triage categories can be assigned:

TRTS	Triage category
1–9	T1
10–11	T2
12	T3
0	T4

Types of triage cards
- Cambridge cruciform; BASICs; METAG; FM (Army)

METHODS OF TRAUMA SCORING (TS)

- Can be physiological, anatomical or a combination

Physiological scoring
- Respiratory rate, respiratory effort, systolic BP, capillary refill time and Glasgow coma scale
- e.g. Revised Trauma Score (see Triage Revised Trauma Score above)
- In the USA a RTS score ≤3 in any one parameter indicates the need for transfer to a level one trauma centre

Anatomical scoring system
- Injury Severity Scale (ISS) is based on the Abbreviated Injury Scale (AIS)
- Each injury is scored from 1 (minor) to 6 (untreatable) using a standard list of injuries
- ISS is the sum of the squares of highest three AIS scores from six body areas (head/neck, face, chest, extremities, abdomen, external, skin

- A score >16 indicates major trauma and an AIS score = 6 in a single area is deemed untreatable and is awarded a score of 75

Anatomical and physiological scoring

- Trauma Score Injury Severity Score (TRISS) combines RTS and ISS with the age of the patient together with the method of injury (blunt or penetrating)

Open fracture grading (ATLS Modification from Gustilo *et al.* and Tscherne *et al.*)[30]

- Grade I – small skin laceration by tip of spiral (indirect) fracture
- Grade II – small-to-moderate, well-circumscribed wound with little contamination and no significant tissue necrosis or periosteal stripping
- Grade IIIa – longer laceration with significant contused or non-viable tissue, but after debridement, delayed suture or split thickness skin graft (STSG) can close the wound
- Grade IIIb – extensive soft tissue wound with crush, contamination and/or periosteal stripping. A local or free muscle flap usually is required to close
- Grade IIIc – an open fracture with a vascular injury that requires repair to salvage the limb
- Grade IV – total or subtotal amputation

COMPARTMENT SYNDROME

Sites of compartment syndrome

- Common
  - Lower leg
  - Forearm
  - Foot
  - Hand
- Uncommon
  - Quadriceps
  - Hamstrings
  - Tensor fascia lata
  - Gluteal muscles
  - Biceps

Mechanism of compartment syndrome

- Reductions in volume, e.g. constricting casts and circumferential burns
- Increase in maximum distensible volume leading to a rise in pressure
- e.g. burns, fractures crush injury, acute muscle tears, post-arterial surgery reperfusion injury, bleeding diathesis, release of surgical tourniquet, pressure due to prolonged anaesthesia, snake bite

Diagnosis of compartment syndrome

- Measure distal oxygen saturation
- Detect reduction in blood using Doppler ultrasound
- Measure intercompartmental pressure

Indications for urgent fasciotomy

- Compartment pressure >50 mmHg
- A rise in compartment pressure to within 30 mmHg of diastolic pressure

SURGERY: FACTS AND FIGURES

COMPLICATIONS OF TRAUMA RESUSCITATION

Technical complications associated with trauma resuscitation[5]

Intervention	Complication(s)
Oesophageal obturator airway	Hypercapnia, tracheal intubation, hypoxia, acidosis
Endotracheal intubation	Oesophageal intubation, traumatic intubation
Positive-pressure breathing	Precipitation of tension pneumothorax air embolism (when associated with lung laceration)
Cutdown intravenous lines	Injury to greater saphenous nerve, injury to median nerve, jury to brachial artery, infection
Percutaneous subclavian central line	Pneumothorax, haemothorax/haemorrhage, infection
Intercostal intubation	Intra-abdominal or diaphragmatic injury, improper placement, retained haemothorax, infection, lung laceration
Diagnostic peritoneal lavage	False-positive/negative lavage, bladder, gastric perforation, bowel or vascular perforation, infection
Arterial lines	Digital ischaemia, infection, local bleeding
MAST suits	Respiratory embarrassment, ?exacerbation of intracranial hypertension, compartment syndrome, limited patient access

SPECIFIC COMPLICATIONS OF ATLS PROCEDURES[30]

Complications of needle cricothyroidotomy

- Asphyxia
- Aspiration
- Cellulitis
- Oesophageal perforation
- Exsanguinating haematoma
- Posterior tracheal wall perforation
- Subcutaneous of mediastinal emphysema
- Thyroid perforation
- Inadequate ventilation leading to hypoxia and death

Complications of a surgical cricothyroidotomy

- Asphyxia
- Aspiration (e.g. blood)
- Cellulitis
- Creation of a false passage
- Subglottic stenosis/oedema
- Laryngeal stenosis
- Haemorrhage or haematoma formation
- Laceration to the oesophagus and trachea
- Mediastinal emphysema
- Vocal cord paralysis, hoarseness

Complications of central venipuncture

- Haematoma formation
- Cellulitis
- Thrombosis
- Phlebitis
- Nerve puncture/transection peripheral neuropathy
- Arterial puncture
- Pneumothorax
- Haemopneumothorax
- Chylothorax
- Arteriovenous fistula
- Lost catheters
- Inaccurate monitoring
- Improper placement of catheters

Complication of femoral punctures

- Haematoma formation
- Cellulitis
- Phlebitis
- Nerve transection or puncture peripheral neuropathy
- Arterial puncture
- Arterio venous fistula formation
- Lost catheters
- Inaccurate monitoring techniques
- Improperly placed catheters

Complications of intraosseous puncture

- Local abscess and cellulitis
- Osteomyelitis
- Sepsis
- Through and through penetration of bone
- Subcutaneous or subperiosteal infiltration
- Pressure necrosis of the skin
- Transient bone marrow hypocellularity
- Physeal plate injury
- Haematoma

Complications of peripheral venous cutdown

- Cellulitis
- Haematoma
- Phlebitis
- Perforation of the posterior wall vein
- Venous thrombosis
- Nerve transection
- Arterial transection

Complications of DPL

- Haemorrhage from operative site
- Peritonitis from bowel perforation

- Perforation of the bladder
- Injury to intra-abdominal or peritoneal structures
- Wound infection

Complications associated with a massive blood transfusion[5]

- Acidosis
- Decreased oxygen delivery
- Hypothermia
- Hypocalcaemia
- Micro-embolization. ?Pulmonary injury
- Dilutional thrombocytopenia
- Coagulopathy
- Disseminated intravascular coagulation (DIC)
- Transfusion reactions

REGIONAL FRACTURES AND TRAUMA

DEFINITIONS

- Subluxation – no longer congruous but loss of contact is not incomplete
- Dislocation – loss of congruity between articulating surfaces of a joint
- Fracture – loss of continuity in the substance of a bone
- Non union – not united in 9 months of injury (if hypertrophic treat by preventing movement; if atrophic bone graft)

GRADES AND TYPES OF DAMAGE

Joint injury[22]

- Subluxation (partial dislocation)
- Dislocation
- Fracture dislocation

Ligament injury[22]

- Sprain, in which stability is maintained
- Partial rupture, in which there is some loss of stability but some fibres remain intact
- Complete rupture, with loss of both stability and continuity of the ligament

Injuries to nerves[22]

- Neurapraxia – transient loss of function caused by outside pressure. Recovery in minutes
- Axonotmesis – loss of function due to more severe compression but without loss of continuity. Recovery in weeks or months
- Neurotmesis – division of the nerve. No recovery unless repaired

PHYSICAL SIGNS OF A FRACTURE[22]

- Abnormal movement in a limb due to movement at the fracture site
- Crepitus or grating between the bone ends
- A deformity that can be seen or felt

- Bruising around the fracture
- Tenderness over the fracture site
- Pain on stressing the limb by bending or longitudinal compression
- Impaired function
- Swelling at the fracture site

FRACTURES THAT MAY BE MISSED[22]

- Impacted fractures of the femoral neck
- Fractures of the ribs
- Fractures of the skull, particularly the base of the skull
- Facial fractures, particularly the zygoma
- Fractures of the radial head
- Fatigue fractures before the callus has appeared
- Fractures of the scaphoid
- Fracture dislocations of the carpus, particularly the lunate
- Seventh cervical vertebra
- Undisplaced fractures of the pelvis
- Fractures of the odontoid
- Fracture dislocation of the tarso-metatarsal joint
- Fracture of the talus

COMPLICATIONS OF FRACTURES[22]

- Early
  - Wound infection
  - Fat embolism
  - Shock lung
  - Chest infection
  - Disseminated intravascular coagulation
  - Exacerbation of generalized illness
- Late
  - Deformity
  - Osteoarthritis of adjacent or distant joints
  - Aseptic necrosis
  - Traumatic chondromalacia
  - Reflex sympathetic dystrophy

BLOOD LOSS FROM COMMON FRACTURES[22]

- Tibia, ankle, elbow, forearm – 1–3 units lost or 0.5–1.5 litres
- Femur, knee, shoulder, humerus – 2–4 units lost or 1–2.5 litres
- Pelvis, hip – 3–5 units lost or 1.5–3 litres

SITES OF AVULSION FRACTURES

- Base of 5th metacarpal – peroneus brevis
- Tibial tuberosity – quadriceps
- Upper pole of patella – quadriceps

- Lesser trochanter – iliopsoas
- Greater tuberosity – supraspinatus

PATHOLOGICAL FRACTURES

A pathological fracture is one that occurs in abnormal bone (usually other than osteoporotic) secondary to normal stresses

Causes of pathological fractures

- Generalized bone disease
  - Osteoporosis
  - Osteogenesis imperfecta
  - Metabolic/endocrine bone disease
    - Hyperparathyroidism
    - Osteomalacia
    - Vitamin C deficiency
    - Cushing's disease
    - Hyperthyroidism
  - Paget's disease
  - Polyostic fibrous dysasia
  - Myelomatosis
  - Endochondromatosis
  - Gaucher's disease
  - Neurofibromatosis
  - Osteopetrosis
- Local benign conditions
  - Chronic infection
  - Solitary bone cyst
  - Fibrous cortical defect
  - Chondromyxoid fibroma
  - Aneurysmal bone cyst
  - Chondroma
  - Monostotic fibrous dysplasia
- Primary malignant bone tumours
  - Chondrosarcoma
  - Osteosarcoma
  - Ewing's tumour
- Metastatic tumours (breast, lung, kidney, thyroid, prostate)

BASIC PRINCIPLES OF FRACTURE MANAGEMENT[21]

- Reduction of the fracture
- Maintenance of the reduction
- Rehabilitation

Rough guide to fracture healing[22]

- Bones join in 8 weeks, but double this in the lower limb and halve it for children

TYPES OF FRACTURE MANAGEMENT[22]

- Splints, slings and casts
- Cast bracing
- Traction
  - Skin or skeletal
  - Fixed or sliding
    - Fixed traction may use splint or gravity
    - Sliding traction may be balanced or not balanced
- External fixation
- Internal fixation

ADVANTAGES AND DISADVANTAGES OF TREATMENT METHODS

Complication of casts[22]

- Circulatory embarrassment
- Pressure sores
- Undiagnosed wound infection
- Joint stiffness

Complications of traction[22]

- Over distraction
- Loss of position
- Pressure sores
- Pin track infection

Advantages of external fixation[22]

- It can be used in patients with skin loss or infection
- Position of the fragments can be easily seen

Main indications for internal fixation[22]

- Fractures that cannot be controlled in any other way
- Patients with fractures of more than one bone
- Fractures in which the blood supply to the limb is jeopardized and the vessels must be protected

Disadvantages of internal fixation[22]

- Risk of infection at the time of operation
- Additional trauma of operation. A wide exposure is needed to apply screws and plates and this must devitalize some of the bone and soft tissue
- There is no virtue in replacing a healthy fracture in almost perfect position with a bone that is anatomically perfect but dead

SKULL FRACTURE

- If minimal and no neurological deficit – leave
- If compound – clean and close

Complications of skull fracture

- Intracranial haematoma
- Cerebrospinal fluid fistula
- Cranial nerve injury
- Cosmetic deformity
- Aerocoele
- Post-concussion syndrome
- Post-traumatic epilepsy
- Meningitis
- Hydrocephalus

MAXILLARY FACIAL FRACTURES

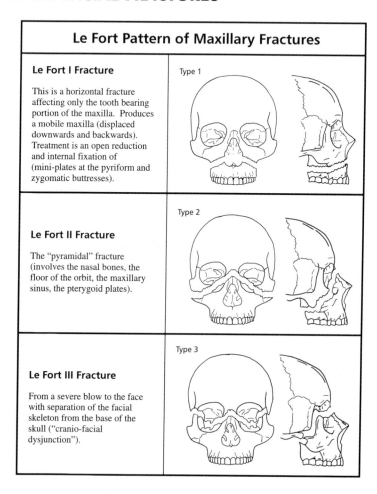

Le Fort Pattern of Maxillary Fractures

Le Fort I Fracture

This is a horizontal fracture affecting only the tooth bearing portion of the maxilla. Produces a mobile maxilla (displaced downwards and backwards). Treatment is an open reduction and internal fixation of (mini-plates at the pyriform and zygomatic buttresses).

Type 1

Le Fort II Fracture

The "pyramidal" fracture (involves the nasal bones, the floor of the orbit, the maxillary sinus, the pterygoid plates).

Type 2

Le Fort III Fracture

From a severe blow to the face with separation of the facial skeleton from the base of the skull ("cranio-facial dysjunction").

Type 3

Figure 14.5 Le Fort classification of maxillary fractures. From: *Sports Medicine: Problems and Practical Management* (Eds E. Sherry & D. Bokor); Greenwich Medical Media, 1997: page 87.

Treatment
- Internal fixators and mini plates

For cervical spine fractures and head injuries, see p XXX

TYPES OF THORACIC FRACTURE[22]

The pattern of fracture depends on the position of the axis of flexion and the direction of the force of impact. The main types are:
- Compression fractures
- Burst fractures
- Seat-belt (flexion/distraction) fractures
- Fracture dislocations

Treatment of vertebral crush fracture
- A wedge fracture is usually stable if the height of the anterior margin is >2/3 the posterior margin
- If the cord is compressed, decompress before traction and stabilization
- Anterior compression
  - <50% – Rx: bed rest if no neurology
  - >50% – Rx: stabilize
- Fragment in spinal canal – Rx – stabilize
- Neurology – Rx – stabilize

Fractured clavicle

Treatment
- Broad arm sling for (2–3 weeks), then mobilize. Bone remodelling takes 2 years
- Non-union (unusual) requires fixation and bone graft
- If malunion of distal third occurs treat like an acromio-clavicular dislocation

Scapular fracture
- Consider underlying lung and rib injuries
- If intra-articular fracture of the glenoid is present perform accurate reduction

Treatment
- Simple sling

SHOULDER DISLOCATION

Types of shoulder dislocation[22]
- Anterior dislocation
- Posterior dislocation
- Luxation erecta, or true inferior dislocation
- Fracture dislocations
- Multidirectional

Methods to reduce the dislocated humeral head[22]
- MUA
- Hanging-arm technique

- Hippocratic method
- Kocher's method

Proximal humeral fracture

- Assess neurovascular and local bony damage
- Fracture of the anatomical neck (rim of articular cartilage) has risk of avascular necrosis (AVN)
- Fracture of surgical neck (area below both tuberosities) causes no AVN but can result in rotator cuff injuries as they attach here therefore unstable fractures should be internally fixed
- Neer
  - 2 part – surgical neck
  - 3 part – head and one tuberosity
  - 4 part – head and both tuberosities. If four part needs Neer's hemiarthroplasty as very painful if treated conservatively

Treatment is related to the Neer classification

- I – all proximal humeral fractures with minimal displacement and irrespective of angulation Manage conservatively collar and cuff
- II – anatomical neck fractures displaced by >1 cm (risk of AVN). Avoid manipulation. Manage conservatively collar and cuff
- III – surgical neck fractures. Displaced or angulated. Manipulate or internally fixate in younger patients, collar and cuff if elderly
- IV – greater tuberosity fractures(supraspinatus insertion, three part). Manage conservatively or Internally fix, depending on size
- V – lesser tuberosity fractures (three or four part) and displacement of bone fragments
- VI – fracture dislocation. If unstable percutaneous pin or internally fixate. If risk of AVN in the elderly perform a hemiarthroplasty

MIDSHAFT HUMERAL FRACTURE[31]

- The Radial nerve is at risk

Treatment

- Collar and cuff and cast brace at 10 days (not a U slab)
- Internally fix – if multiple injury (more than two fractures), non-union, radial nerve involvement, or if in an unacceptable position after:
  - Trial of conservative therapy
  - Using dynamic compression plate, Kuntschner nail, Rush pin (solid intermedullary nails with hooked ends)
- Complications – radial nerve injury in closed injuries due to neuropraxia. 90% will recover

SUPRA CONDYLAR FRACTURE[31]

- Causes disruption of elbow function and carries a risk of injuring the median or ulnar nerve brachial artery and can result in a varus deformity (gunstock reversal of carrying angle), Volkman's ischaemic contracture (pain on passive extension and flexion) joint stiffness, traction neuritis, myositis ossificans, or hypertrophic bone formation

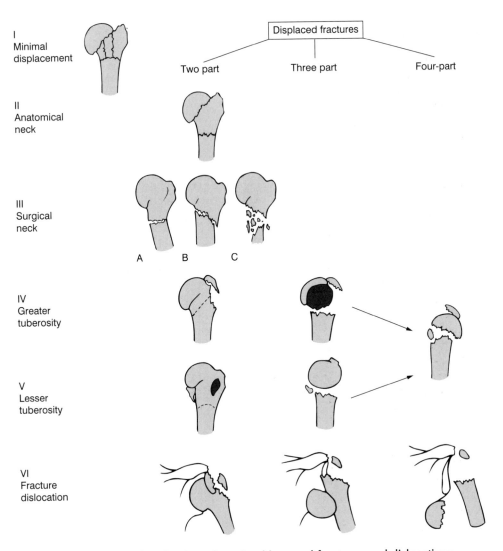

I
Minimal
displacement

Displaced fractures

Two part   Three part   Four-part

II
Anatomical
neck

III
Surgical
neck

A   B   C

IV
Greater
tuberosity

V
Lesser
tuberosity

VI
Fracture
dislocation

Figure 14.6 Neer's classification of proximal humeral fractures and dislocations.

Treatment

Reduce if:

- Neurovascular injury
- Backward tilting of >15°, i.e. <30° (normal range 45°)
- Lateral tilting of >10° (normal range 10°)
- Lateral/medial displacement of >50%
- In children lateral angulation >20° if cannot manipulate reduce via traction on coronoid process

Note: if a fracture or dislocation has been missed still try to reduce up to 6 weeks post-injury

DISLOCATION OF THE ELBOW[31]

Treatment

- Reduction under anaesthesia and in view of the soft tissue damage POP immobilization
- Complications – injury to the brachial artery, Compartment syndrome, neuropraxia to median or ulnar nerves, myositis ossificans with secondary loss of function, redislocation due to gross disruption of ligament and capsule

FRACTURE OF MEDIAL EPICONDYLE[31]

Treatment

- Undisplaced – manage conservatively with regular radiological review
- Displaced – require accurate reduction and may require fixation with K wires
- Complications – ulnar nerve palsy, varus deformity due to growth arrest, pain and stiffness

FRACTURES OF THE CAPITELLUM[31]

Treatment

- Open reduction is the treatment of choice using Herbert screws and early mobilization

FRACTURES OF LATERAL CONDYLE[31]

Treatment

- Undisplaced – POP with forearm pronated and elbow at 90°. Regular radiological review as prone to slippage
- Displaced – accurate manipulation and fixation with K wires or open reduction
- Complications – malunion, growth arrest with deformity, ulnar nerve palsy

FRACTURES OF THE OLECRANON[31]

- Olecranon forms the insertion point of extensors. If undisplaced it implies that the triceps can function

Treatment

- Undisplaced – short-term plaster immobilization and observation to exclude displacement
- Displaced – reconstitute triceps mechanism using open reduction and fixation usually with K wires and a tension band
- Compound – debridement and consideration of early fixation. using plates and screws (Zuelzer hooked plate, Croll olecranon screw, lag screw, contour plate)

HEAD OF RADIUS FRACTURE[31]

- Fat pad effusion apparent on radiograph. If intra-articular, it can result in major stiffness and disability

Treatment

- Undisplaced – aspiration of haemarthrosis, instillation of local anaesthetic, after initial rest, mobilize in a collar and cuff with physiotherapy

- Displaced and intra-articular – fixed with a Herbert screw (no prominent head and differential pitch compresses fracture) or removed (and replaced with a spacer) with POP for 2/52
- Comminuted – radial head can be excised acutely and a short-term silastic spacer is inserted to prevent radial shortening, cubitus valgus deformity and resulting complications, e.g. ulnar nerve palsy. The spacer is removed at 6 months

If diagnosis is delayed there is often a function block to flexion, which will be improved by excision of the fragments. In rare cases a large single fragment may be reduced and fixed.

RADIUS AND ULNA FRACTURE[31]

- The radius rolls over the ulna to allow pronation (palm downwards) and supination
- Radial bowing and intact joints are necessary for normal function
- If one bone of the forearm is fractured the other is always fractured or dislocated:
    - Monteggia – fractured ulna, dislocated proximal radius
    - Galeazzi – fractured radius, dislocated distal ulna

Treatment

- Open reduction and plating as otherwise the complication of delayed union is relatively common
- Remove at 18 months if young but beware injuring posterior interosseous nerve 1–2 cm below radial neck

WRIST FRACTURES[31]

Colles' fracture/Treatment

- Stable
- Single undisplaced extra-articular – back slab with completion of plaster after 24 or 48 h when soft tissue swelling is resolving. Maintain immobilization for 5 weeks in ulnar deviated cast then mobilize
- Displaced extra-articular – Charnley reduction and three-point Colles' plaster for 5 weeks
- Manipulate if:
    - >10° Dorsal tilt (the normal position is 5° forward)
    - Fracture of ulnar styloid
    - Radius displacement and disruption of the inferior radio ulnar joint
    - Radial impaction(not out to length)
- Unstable
- Dorsal angulation of 20°or more
- Extensive intrarticular involvement
- Comminution of dorsal surface (leads to loss of position)
- If articular and young, treat by external fixation, bone graft, internally fix or a combination
- If comminuted, treat by external fixation. Insert K wires or the Pennig fixator which has the advantage of allowing early mobilization
- Complications – stiff wrist, 10% functional deformity, median N compression, rupture of EPL, reflex sympathetic dystrophy (Rx aggressive physiotherapy and guanethidine blockade of sympathetic NS)

Smith's fracture

- A reversed Colles

Treatment

Due to inherent instability treat by open reduction and internal fixation with a volar plate

Barton's fracture

- A partial Smith's in which only anterior part of radius is fractured
- If cannot be reduced use T plate, cancellous screws or an Ellis buttress plate

HAND INJURIES[31]

Scaphoid fracture

- The Scaphoid is the keystone of the wrist. The most common fractures are of the waist of the scaphoid and are managed in a scaphoid plaster for 6 weeks

Treatment

- If acute and displaced, stabilize with a Herbert screw which compresses as at different pitches
- Complications – Sudeck's atrophy, non-union (graft). Proximal pole prone to malunion assess with MRI

FRACTURED HOOK OF HAMATE

Treatment if symptomatic

- Excise

CARPEL DISLOCATION

- Most common patterns are Lunate, perilunate dislocation and scapho-lunate dislocation

Treatment

- Reduce and maintain reduction for 4 weeks

DISLOCATED LUNATE

- Diagnosed if radius, lunate, capitate, and fifth metacarpel are not in line
- Complications – acute median nerve compression and AVN (Kleinbock's disease) perform check radiograph at 6 months

METACARPAL FRACTURES

- Fracture of the neck of the fifth metacarpal (Boxer's fracture)

Treatment

- Early mobilization by neighbour strapping
- Exceptionally operative intervention may be required, e.g. in pianists

SPIRAL FRACTURES

- Rarely lead to any significant functionally loss

Treatment

- If multiple or without angulation treat with volar slab with the metacarpophalangeal joints flexed to 90° and interphalangeal joints to 180° (the position of function) for 7–10 days
- Significant angulation or rotational deformity often requires internal fixation for correct alignment

PHALANGEAL FRACTURES

Treatment

- Neighbour strapping or volar slab in the position of function
- Transverse fractures are prone to angulation and spiral fractures are prone to rotation during the first 10 days and require frequent follow-up. Failure to maintain correct position indicates open reduction and fixation
- Fractures involving the interphalangeal joints often lead to residual stiffness and should be considered for reduction and fixation

DISLOCATIONS

- Most of these injuries can be reduced after administration of a ring block
- However if 'button holing' through the ligaments, capsule or volar plate occurs open reduction and repair may be required

OPEN INJURIES OF THE HAND

- Lacerations
  - Superficial or deep
  - Clean or contaminated
- Foreign bodies
- Motor deficit
  - Extensor tendon injury
  - Flexor tendon injury
- Nerve damage – sensory loss
- Note patient handedness

Treatment

- Clean wound
- Remove foreign body and debris
- Asses tendon damage
- Extensor tendon – primary repair
- Flexor tendon
  - Primary suture only if wound clean and early operation
  - Laceration with in flexor sheath may require secondary suture and grafting (between distal palmar crease and proximal interphalangeal joint – risk of adhesions)
- Antibiotics

- Splintage with flexed metacarpophalangeal joint
- Elevation
- Early mobilization

SITES OF FLEXOR TENDON INJURY[22]

- Zone I – distal to d.i.p. joint
- Zone II – in the fingers
- Zone III – in the palm
- Zone IV – in the carpal tunnel
- Zone V – in the forearm

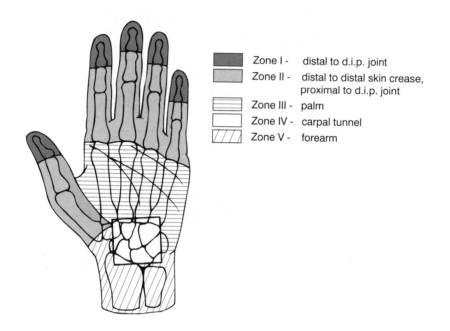

Zone I - distal to d.i.p. joint
Zone II - distal to distal skin crease, proximal to d.i.p. joint
Zone III - palm
Zone IV - carpal tunnel
Zone V - forearm

Figure 14.7 Flexor tendon zones in the hand.

LOWER BODY

PELVIC FRACTURE

- Take Judet views, iliac and obturator obliques to show anterior and posterior columns
- Conservative Treatment – bed rest for 6–8 weeks, non-weight-bearing for 10–12 weeks, insert fenestrated catheter. Note: check sacroiliac joints
- Operative Treatment
  - Anterior column – use Semitubular plate
  - Posterior column – use Sacral bars

Note: if unstable and exsanguinating, treat by emergency external fixation (priority before laparotomy) or use arteriography with embolization

Acetabular fracture

- Can result in long-term degeneration; therefore need accurate reduction and fixation in specialist units

Ischial tuberosity

- Treatment – fixation

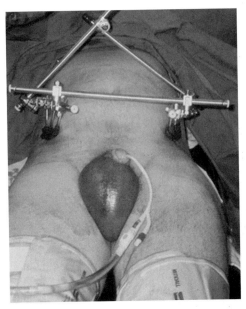

Figure 14.8 External fixator applied to unstable 'open book' pelvic fracture. From: *Sports Medicine: Problems and Practical Management* (Eds E. Sherry & D. Bokor); Greenwich Medical Media, 1997.

HIP DISLOCATIONS[31]

- 85% are posterior after trauma

Anterior dislocation

- Associated neurovascular injury may occur, after reduction maintain on traction for 6 weeks

Posterior dislocation

- Epstein classification of posterior dislocations
- Type I – dislocation with minor chip fracture
- Type II – dislocation with single large posterior fragment
- Type III – dislocation with comminution of the posterior acetabular lip
- Type IV – dislocation with associated fracture of the acetabular floor
- Type V – dislocation with fracture of the head of the femur

Rx

- Type I injuries – 3 weeks of traction

- All others require 6 weeks of traction post-reduction
- Operative treatment is indicated if:
- Intra-articular fragments are present
- Epstein Type II injury
- Epstein type IV and V injuries (if spontaneous reduction does not occur on hip relocation)

COMPLICATIONS OF POSTERIOR DISLOCATION OF THE HIP[22]

- Damage to the sciatic nerve – the lateral part of the sciatic nerve responsible for the dorsi-flexion of the foot lies immediately behind the hip and is often damaged in posterior fracture dislocation
- Aseptic necrosis of the femoral head – aseptic necrosis of the femoral head occurs in ~20% of patients with this injury but the incidence is less if the hip is reduced soon after injury. Aseptic necrosis may not be apparent until 2 years or, in exceptional cases, 8 years later. This is important when assessing long-term prognosis of the injury necessary for legal purposes if the fracture occurred in a road accident
- Osteoarthritis – if the femoral head has been damaged or there is aseptic necrosis, osteoarthritis is almost inevitable
- Ectopic ossification can occur round a dislocated hip, reducing joint movement and causing pain

FRACTURED NECK OF FEMUR[31]

Femoral neck fractures

- Risk factors
  - Elderly
  - Women
  - Osteoporosis
- Clinical Features
  - History of fall or twist
  - Limb in lateral rotation and shortened
- Classification
- Gardens':
  - Stage I – incomplete (impacted, not full width of neck involved)
  - Stage II – complete neck fracture, no displacement
  - Stage III – complete neck fracture with partial displacement
  - Stage IV – complete neck fracture with full displacement, posterior retinacular attachment no longer connected
- Treatment
  - Elderly
    - High risk of avascular necrosis of femoral head
    - Hemiarthroplasty with metal prosthesis
  - Young – open reduction, transfemoral screw fixation
  - Children
    - Undisplaced – plaster cast until united
    - Displaced – reduction and pin or screw fixation

Note: in the Garden classification grades III and IV the blood supply is interrupted.

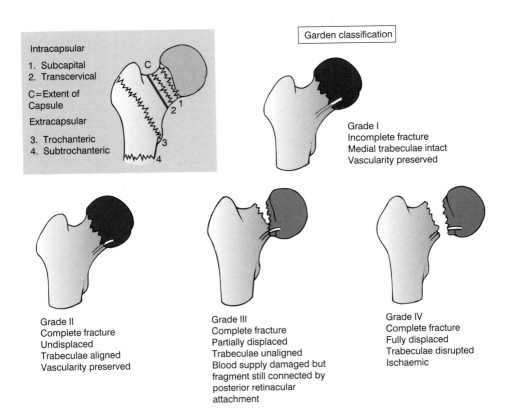

Figure 14.9 Types and grading of proximal femoral fractures. Note: in Garden Classification grades II and IV, the blood supply is interrupted.

INTRATROCHANTERIC (EXTRACAPSULAR) FRACTURES

Treatment
- 'Dynamic hip screw' whether stable or unstable

Isolated trochanteric fractures
- Occur at the lesser trochanter caused by the pull of the psoas muscle and the greater trochanter due to the pull of the abductor muscle

Treatment
- Rest, pain relief and early mobilization

FEMORAL NECK (HIP) FRACTURE[31]

Need to differentiate intracapsular with their high risk of AVN from extracapsular fractures

- Type I – inferior cortex only <70 years pin/screw Contraindications: steroids, >48 h post injury
- Type II – complete fracture not displaced 20–30% risk of AVN
- Type III – slight displacement
- Type IV – fully displaced
- If >70 years, Austin Moore (no cement) Thompson's (cement) hemiarthroplasty

INTRACAPSULAR

- Subcapital or trancervical (risk AVN) relate to biological age and expected functional outcome
- If young age and undisplaced try parallel cannulated screw, Garden nails
- If elderly hemiarthroplasty (Thompson, Austin Moore) or THR

EXTRACAPSULAR OR TROCHANTERIC

- No AVN, but a tendency to collapse into varus with a risk of shortening and malunion
- Medial femoral neck and upper shaft form a medial buttress which is critical for stability
- Avulsion of the lesser trochanter indicates comminution of this area and implies instability
- These injuries, like all cancellous fractures, heal by impaction – therefore use DHS which allows screw to slide back towards the plate accommodating the collapse
- Post-DHS, many do not survive 6/12

Note: non-operative treatment does not usually lead to death but to dependency.

Subtrochanteric

- Often pathological – blade plate or interlocking intermedullary nail and treat primary cause

FRACTURE OF THE SHAFT OF THE FEMUR[31]

- High energy injury

Treatment

- Intermedullary nailing with distal and proximal locking to maintain length and prevents relative rotation of the proximal and distal parts of the femur
- Complications – early shock and fat embolism, intermediate thromboembolism, late delayed union, malunion and non-union

FEMORAL CONDYLAR FRACTURE[31]

Treatment

- If intra-articular open reduction, fixation and rehabilitation
- Need exact intrarticular congruency therefore use a dynamic condylar screw

PATELLA FRACTURE[31]

- If comminuted but enclosed without disruption of lateral patella retinaculum – Rx: plaster and gentle, passive movements

- If loss of quadriceps mechanism – Rx: surgical stabilization; tension band wiring if multiple small fragments which are difficult to reconstruct – patellectomy

KNEE JOINT INJURIES[21]

Anterior cruciate rupture
Treatment

- Jones reconstruction uses 1/3 of the patella tendon whereas MacIntosh utilizes fascia lata

FRACTURES OF THE TIBIAL PLATEAU[31]
Treatment

- Open reduction and buttress plating with or without bone grafting is the treatment of choice to restore the joint surface and have an early restoration of function. The exceptions are undisplaced fractures and in the elderly where conservative treatment usually suffices
- Complications – compartment syndrome, malunion and secondary osteoarthritis

FRACTURES OF THE SHAFTS OF THE TIBIA[31]

- Classification – transverse, oblique, spiral
- Unacceptable fracture displacement
  - Shortening >1 cm
  - >50% lateral shift
  - >5% varus/valgus
  - >10% anterior or posterior (anterior is especially distressing)

Treatment

- Best treated with intramedullary nailing with proximal and distal locking
- Isolated fibular shaft fractures are treated in below-knee plasters
- Complications
  - Neurovascular injury
  - Compartment syndrome
  - Infection (in compound fractures nailing should follow wound debridement)
  - Delayed union, malunion non-union
  - Inadequate skin cover and healing (liase with plastic surgeons)
  - Ankle and knee joint stiffness

MAISSONUEUVE FRACTURE

- A fracture of the proximal fibula with diastasis of the distal talofibular joint and subluxation of the talus

Treatment

- Cerclage

INJURIES TO THE ANKLE[22]

- The ankle is supported by a complex ring of bone and ligaments. A fracture of one part of the ring thus implies fracture of another part

SURGERY: FACTS AND FIGURES

- Bones may be broken in the ankle at three points:
  - Medial malleolus of the tibia
  - Lower end of the fibula, including the lateral malleolus
  - 'Posterior malleolus, or posterior margin of the tibia
- Three ligaments may be torn:
  - Inferior tibiofibular ligament
  - Medial ligament
  - Lateral collateral ligament
- Four forces may contribute to the injury:
  - Abduction
  - Adduction
  - External rotation
  - Vertical compression
- Five grades of severity are seen:
  - Ligament injury alone
  - Ligament injury plus one malleolus
  - Ligament injury plus two malleoli
  - Ligament injury plus all three malleoli
  - Ligament injury plus diastasis of the inferior tibiofibular joint plus fracture

Fracture management

- The aim is to establish a stable mortise
- To assess the degree of damage to malleoli, medial and lateral ligaments, and the interosseous membrane
- Later degenerative changes are related to the quality of the reduction

Classification of ankle fractures

- Weber (1972)
  - A – below the level of the syndesmoses (the distal tibio fibular joint)
  - B – at below the level of the syndesmoses (spiral fractures beginning at the level of the plafond and extending proximally)
  - C – above below the level of the syndesmoses and interosseous torn

Note: types B and C are invariably unstable and are likely to need orthopaedic intervention

- Potts – one malleolar, bimalleolar or three (including inferior arcticular surface of the tibia)
- Lauge-Hanson (most useful classification in assessing prognosis)
  - Supintion-adduction
  - Supination-eversion
  - Pronation-abduction
  - Pronation-eversion

Treatment

- Close reduction for:
  - Anatomical and able to be held without repeated manipulations
  - Operation contraindicated due to the general condition of patient or the fracture is undisplaced and stable
  - Grossly comminuted fractures (use conservative traction of 2 kg via a calcaneal pin)
  - Osteoarthritis can result

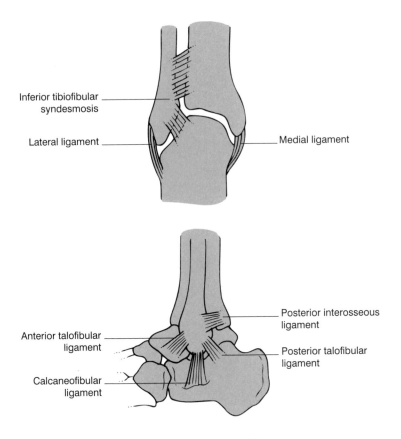

Figure 14.10 Structures that may be injured at the ankle.

- Open reduction for:
  - Failure of closed reduction
  - If closed reduction requires abnormal positioning of foot
  - Fracture/ankle is displaced or unstable
  - (A displaced medial malleolus usually has soft tissue interposition: periosteum, extensor retinaculum or posterior tibialis)
  - Stability is to be guaranteed
- Window of opportunity for open reduction is at <8 h or after 5–7 days, before swelling begins or after it has subsided

Note: fix fibula before medial malleolus and if cross screws are used to correct the diastasis do so in dorsiflexion (otherwise this movement will be restricted). Studies show that patients who have early fixation and movement return to work sooner, have no radiological signs of OA but spend longer in hospital.

DISRUPTED SYNDESMOSES

Treatment

- Controversial
- If intraoperative assessment shows instability syndesmotic screw can be inserted with the foot dorsiflexed
- Plaster splint elevate for 24–48 h with a cast for 6 weeks

OTHER LIGAMENTOUS INJURY

- Immobilization of severe grade III lateral collateral ligament injuries is sometimes undertaken in athletes and re-routing of the tendon of peroneus brevis occasionally occurs

TALAR FRACTURES[31]

- Usually due to forced dorsiflexion and are prone to vascular complications. The blood supply is via the anterior tibial, posterior tibial and peroneal vessels
- Hawkins' classification defines the amount of additional soft tissue damage and hence the risk of AVN
  - Type I – undisplaced through talar neck (only one source of blood supply is compromised)
  - Type II – fracture with subluxation or dislocation of subtalar joint (at least two sources are compromised)
  - Type III – fracture with dislocation of subtalar and ankle joints (all sources of blood supply are lost)
  - Types II and III require early reduction and internal fixation
- Undisplaced – POP with foot plantigraded for 8 weeks. The plaster is not weight-bearing in fractures of the neck and the body but is weight-bearing in fractures of the head
- Displaced and fracture dislocations
  - Attempt closed reduction by forced plantar flexion with immobilization for 2–3 weeks in plaster in plantar flexion followed by 6–8 weeks in neutral position, but this often fails and will require open fixation with lag screws. Large, bony fragments from the body or head (dome) require open fixation
  - Dislocations require prompt reduction to prevent skin damage
  - Compound fractures require surgical debridement and delayed primary closure or grafting

Complications

- Skin damage
- Avascular necrosis in approximately 50% of talar neck fractures (many will have reasonable function if protected from weight-bearing)
- Malunion that predisposes to secondary osteoarthrosis

CALCANEAL FRACTURES[31]

- Most are intra-articular affecting the subtalar joint and are caused by a fall from height. Often cause a D-shaped haematoma on the sole. Primary and secondary fracture lines generated by the talus cleave the calcaneus from above

- Essex–Lopresti classification is based on the appearance of the fracture line on the lateral radiograph
  - Tongue type – fracture runs through the body posteriorly, ending below the insertion of the Achilles' tendon
  - Joint depression fragment – a secondary fracture line passes down to the lateral side of the calcaneum behind the posterior articular facet
- Eastwood based a classification system on the coronal CT appearances of the lateral wall for patients undergoing operative intervention
  - Type I – lateral wall is formed solely by the lateral joint fragment
  - Type II – lateral wall is formed by the lateral joint fragment superiorly and the body fragment inferiorly
  - Type III – lateral wall is formed solely by the body fragment
- Displacement is determined by measuring Bohler' angle

Treatment

- Displaced avulsions are reduced and fixed followed by 4–6-week immobilization in a weight-bearing plaster
- Extra-articular fractures RICE, a non-weight-bearing plaster and crutches for 6 weeks
- Intra-articular fractures
  - Undisplaced or minimally displaced as treated like extra-articular fractures
  - Displaced open reduction and internal fixation (grafting where required) followed by a non-weight-bearing plaster for 8 weeks

Complications

- Skin blistering, malunion (usually valgus with a broad heel), peroneal tendon infringement due to the valgus heel. Fibular abutment (fibula catches on the side of the calcaneum). Stiffness and secondary osteoarthritis (if significant subtalar arthrodesis produces the most satisfactory results)

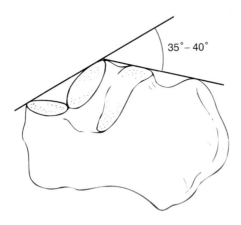

Figure 14.11 Bohler's angle of the calcaneum.

FOOT FRACTURES[31]

Treatment of midtarsal and tarso-metatarsal injuries

- Undisplaced
  - Minor fractures – rest, ice, compression and elevation (RICE)
  - POP immobilization for 4–6 weeks may be necessary
- Displaced – open reduction and internal fixation should be considered
- Fracture dislocations – closed manipulation or open reduction with K wiring
- Lisfranc dislocation (diastasis between the first and second metatarsal)
- If the longitudinal arch of the foot is lost, surgical stabilization is required. If the arch remains and displacement is minimal conservative treatment produces similar results

METATARSAL INJURY

Shaft fractures and crush injuries

- RICE, immobilization a double tubigrip or walking plaster
- Marked displacement – closed manipulation. Open reduction and K wiring may be indicated especially in fractures of the first ad third metatarsals

Base of fifth metatarsal

- Undisplaced light support or weight bearing plaster or ~6 weeks
- If distal to inferior metatarsal joint (Jones' stress fracture)

March fractures

- Double tubigrip; if pain is severe below-knee walking plaster

Metataso-phalangeal injuries

- Dislocations are treated in a light-weight-bearing cast for 4 weeks

Phalangeal fractures

- RICE if there is no displacement or compound injury. Occasionally closed manipulation of angulated fractures is required

Sesamoid fractures

- RICE occasionally immobilization is required for symptomatic relief

NERVE INJURIES

- Closed – can be expected to recover if in continuity
- Open
  - Primary repair within 24 h
  - Secondary with 7-day neuroma resected and gap bridged
- Poor prognosis – complete lesions pain, Horner's, meningocoeles – root avulsion, preganglionic

MANAGEMENT OF BRACHIAL PLEXUS LESIONS[22]

- Identify the site of the lesion by careful neurological examination and EMG
- Decide if the lesion is pre- or postganglionic

- Preganglionic lesions cannot be repaired – absent axonal reflex. Histamine test is positive, Horner's syndrome)
- Postganglionic lesions have a better prognosis. The more distal, the better the outlook
- Surgical repair or grafting is sometimes possible for clean cuts and distal lesions

Examples

- C5, 6 lesion (Erb's palsy) – waiters' tip
- C8, T1 lesion (Klumpke's palsy) – all the muscles of hand and fingers are paralysed, therefore a claw hand due to intrinsic muscular paralysis
- If the sympathetic trunk is involved, Horner's syndrome will occur

ASSESSMENT OF THE PERIPHERAL NERVES

Upper extremities

Nerve	Motor	Sensation
Upper extremities		
Ulnar	Index finger abduction	Little finger
Median-distal	Thenar contraction with opposition	Index finger
Median-ant. interosseous	Index tip flexion	–
Musculocutaneous	Elbow flexion	Lateral forearm
Radial	Thumb extension/abduction	Dorsal web between thumb and index finger
Axillary	Deltoid contraction with shoulder abduction	Lateral shoulder
Lower extremities		
Femoral	Knee extension	Anterior knee
Obturator	Hip adduction	Medial thigh
Tibial	Toe flexion	Sole of foot
Superficial peroneal	Ankle eversion	Lateral dorsum of foot
Deep peroneal space	Ankle/toe dorsiflexion	Dorsal first to second toe
Superior gluteal	Hip adduction	–
Inferior gluteal	Gluteus maximus contraction with hip extension	–

TRAUMA IN CHILDREN

NORMAL VALUES OF COMMONLY MEASURED PARAMETERS IN THE CHILD

Age (years)	Respiratory rate (breaths/min)	Pulse rate (beats/min)	Systolic blood pressure (mmHg)
Newborn	–	160	60–80
< 1	30–40	110–160	70–90
1–5	25–30	95–140	80–100
6–12	20–25	80–120	90–110
> 13	–	60–100	100–120

GLASGOW COMA SCORE

See page 325.

SPINAL CORD INJURY IN CHILDREN

- Are less common than in adults
- Account for <5% of all spinal injuries
- Two-thirds of children with cervical spinal injuries have normal X-rays

DIFFERENCES BETWEEN A CHILD'S AND ADULTS CERVICAL SPINE

- Interspinous ligaments and joint capsules are more flexible
- Uncinate articulations are poorly developed and incomplete
- Vertebral bodies are wedged anteriorly and have a tendency to slide forward with flexion
- Facet joints are flat
- Radiologically
    - Anterior displacement (pseudo-subluxation) of C2 or C3 (less common C3–C4) occurs in 40% of the under 7 age group and in 20% of the under 16 age group
    - In 20% of children there is an increased gap between the dens and the anterior arch of C1
    - Basal odontoid epiphysis may resemble fractures in the under 5 age group; apical odontoid epiphysis may resemble fracture between the ages of 5 and 11
    - Secondary ossification centre at the tip of spinous processes may resemble a fracture

EPIPHYSEAL FRACTURES

- Weakest point is where cartilage hypertrophies. The active region remains with epiphysis

ELBOW INJURIES CHILDREN[31]

- Supracondylar

Treatment

- Undisplaced – immobilization <90°. If flexion causes loss of pulses the arm is extended until these reappear. If this position does not maintain reduction the arm may be mobilized in Dunlop traction

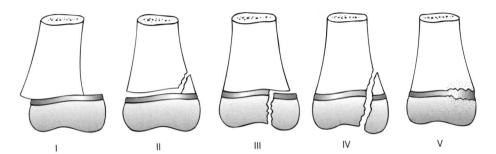

Figure 14.12 Salter and Harris classification of epiphyseal injuries. I, epiphyseal slip only (with no fracture!); II, Fracture through the epiphyseal plate with a triangular fragment of shaft attached to the epiphysis; III, Fracture through the epiphysis extension to the epiphyseal plate; IV, Fracture through the epiphysis and shaft crossing the epiphyseal plate; V, crush injury causing obliteration of the epiphyseal plate which can lead to arrested growth.

- Displaced – reduction under GA, then immobilization. If pulses are not present post-reduction surgical exploration may be necessary. If unstable, open reduction and K wiring may be needed
- Complications
  - Brachial artery injury
  - Compartment syndrome
  - Neuropraxia to the median nerve
  - Malunion with loss of carrying angle and gunstock deformity
  - Volkman's ischaemic contraction
  - Myositis ossificans

PULLED ELBOW[31]

Treatment
- Reduce by swift pronation of the forearm with compression along the radius. A clunk should be felt. If no normal function has occurred after 1 h exclude a fracture radiologically

FEMORAL NECK FRACTURES IN CHILDREN[31]

- Rare

Rx
- Undisplaced – treat conservatively
- Displaced – closed reduction and fixation with hip screw

LONG BONE FRACTURES IN CHILDREN[31]

- Fracture healing is modified by the pliability of the growing bones. Generally most fractures are treated conservatively unless growth plates or articular surfaces are involved with the exception of forearm fractures which are plated to prevent rotational deformity

NON ACCIDENTAL INJURY (NAI) OF CHILDREN[31]

- Risk factors
  - Birth weight <2500 g
  - Mother aged <30 years
  - Unwanted pregnancy
  - Marital stress
  - Lower socio-economic class
- Suggestive signs
  - Inappropriate delay or failure to seek medical advice
  - Vague or inconsistent history, or injury not consistent with the injury
  - Inappropriate parental reaction
    - Lack of concern
    - Hostility to questioning
    - Attempt to leave before consultation is complete
  - Inappropriate reaction of child to parents
  - Failure to thrive
  - Child volunteers that carer or parent caused the injury
  - Previous injury to the child or sibling
- Common injuries in NAI
  - Bruising to face
  - Finger-shaped bruising
  - Linear bruising
  - Burns particularly from cigarettes
  - Abrasions
  - Bruises of different ages
  - Subconjuctival haemorrhages
  - Hyphaema
  - Bulging fontanelle
  - Adult human bite marks
  - Torn frenulum
- Radiological features suggestive of NAI
  - Any fracture in a child <3 years
  - Metaphyseal flake fractures of long bones
  - Spiral fractures of long bones in infants
  - Fractures with epiphyseal displacement
  - Multiple rib fractures on CXR
  - Multiple fractures of different ages on skeletal survey
- Healing fractures suggesting delay in seeking medical advice

15

SURGICAL OUTCOMES

AUDIT
RESEARCH
LAW
ETHICS
CRITERIA FOR A SURGEON

AUDIT

- Clinical audit is defined by the Department of Health (1989) as 'The systematic, critical analysis of the quality of medical care, including the procedures used for diagnosis, and treatment, to help to provide reassurance that the best quality of service is being achieved, having regard to the resources available'
- Medical audit usually refers to assessment by peer review of the medical care provided by the medical profession
- Clinical audit refers to an assessment of the total care of the patient by nurses and professions allied to medicine
- Audit has much in common with resource management as it aims to achieve more effective use of resources, but so far £48 million allocated for audit by the Department of Health in 1991 has as yet failed to demonstrate any value for money
- Managers are especially interested in the use of audit as quality standards and outcome measures are specified in contracts

IMPLEMENTATION OF CHANGE AND CLOSING THE 'AUDIT LOOP'

- For audit to be effective it must lead to beneficial change
- The audit cycle is the comparison between observed practice and the normal standard
- Practice is then changed to improve standards and to re-audited to see if this change provides improvement
- This is termed closing the 'Audit loop'

WHAT AUDIT CAN ASSESS

- Structure – quantity, type of resources
- Process – what is done to the patient
- Outcome – result of clinical intervention

AUDIT TYPES

- Basic clinical audit
- Case type, complications, morbidity and mortality
- Contrast with previous time, different firm, other hospital
- Incident review – critical incidences, resuscitation, leaking AAA, emergency IVU use
- Outcome audit – result of clinical intervention
- Clinical record review – random case note selection (medico-legal education)
- Criterion audit – waiting time, investigations ordered outcome
- Adverse outcome screening – wound infection, risk management, trends
- Focused audit – specific outcome/research
- National studies – CEPOD reviewed deaths within 30 days of an operative procedure and it was concerned with prophylaxis against surgical complications, resuscitation, operations, when to call senior help, head injuries, diabetes management, problems with elderly, records and local anaesthetic

DIFFERENCE BETWEEN AUDIT AND RESEARCH

- Research defines best practice (therefore best care) whereas audit determines whether good care is being practised given the resources
- Audit has a valuable educational component and can be used identify areas for research

RESEARCH[34]

Any research project should begin with an hypothesis. The experiment is then designed to disprove the hypothesis and statistical testing is carried out to assess whether a difference is produced as a result of any intervention. Because the experiment should attempt to disprove the main hypothesis, the assumption is made that there is, in fact, no difference between the groups and that any apparent difference between them occurred by chance. This is called the null hypothesis. Statistical tests are designed to show whether any difference between the groups could have occurred by chance. This is expressed as probability (p). $p = 0.5$ means that the result obtained will occur by chance on 50% of the occasions on which the test is repeated and, therefore, that there is no difference between the groups. $p = 0.05$ means that the result obtained will occur by chance only once in every 20 times the test is repeated and by convention is not a chance finding. This is commonly expressed in the statement that the result is 'statistically significant'. However, statistical significance does not necessarily mean clinical importance. 'A difference is only a difference if it makes a difference.'

SELECTING THE RIGHT STATISTICAL METHOD[34]

Appropriate statistical tests for given data sets

Type of data	Normal	Non-parametric or small numbers
Comparison of two independent groups		
• Interval	Unpaired t-test	Mann–Whitney U test
• Ordinal	Mann–Whitney U test	
• Nominal, with order	Chi square test	
• Nominal, without order	Chi square test	
• Dichotomous	Fisher's exact test	
Comparison of same group under different conditions		
• Interval	Paired t-test	Wilcoxon signed rank test
• Ordinal or nominal	Sign test	
• Dichotomous		Matched pairs test (McNemar or Liddell)
Relationship between two groups		
• Interval versus interval	Simple linear regression; or Pearson's product moment	Linear regression; Kendall's or Spearman rank correlation
• Interval versus ordinal or nominal	One-way analysis of variance	Kruskal–Wallis test
• Ordinal versus ordinal		Kendall's or Spearman rank correlation

Note:
Interval data have a scale with fixed and defined intervals, e.g. time or temperature. *Ordinal data* are arranged in scores from low through to high, e.g. pain scores on a visual analogue scale. *Nominal data with order* are arranged in discrete categories but with some order imposed, e.g. mild, moderate, severe. It can be difficult to distinguish from ordinal data. *Nominal data without order* are arranged in discrete categories, e.g. blood group. *Dichotomous data* comprises two distinct categories.

CRITICAL READING[34]

Some system for deciding the quality of evidence presented in any published report is necessary. Certain standard questions should be asked about any published study:

- Is the study of any clinical importance?
- Is the population from which the study subjects were drawn well defined? Is the sample used representative of the population?
- Are the inclusion/exclusion criteria clearly defined and are they satisfactory? Is the sample size adequate?
- What happened to refusers/dropouts?
- Are the data from the refusers/dropouts included in the report? Are concurrent controls used?
- Is the method of allocation to treatment groups described and is it satisfactory? Is the treatment well defined?
- Are the outcome criteria clearly defined?
- Were the organizers and patients blinded about which treatment the patients were receiving?

These questions allow judgements to be made about the reliability and significance of a study. If the answers are satisfactory the evidence from that study can then be weighed against the evidence from other sources to determine the appropriate clinical action.

LAW

- Consent is based on the ethical principle that 'Every human being of adult years and sound mind has a right to determine what shall be done with his own body'. To protect this autonomy it is a doctor's duty to obtain a patient's consent for the purpose of diagnosis and treatment. Equally important is the patient's right of refusal which should be respected

FORMS OF CONSENT

Expressed

- There are various types of consent. It does not have to be in a written form though documentation is important (especially if verbal) as it will be easier to argue later that consent had been obtained

Implied

- The law recognizes that in some cases the patient's conduct implies his state of mind, e.g. standing in a queue and then holding up an arm for vaccination is 'as clear assent as if it were expressed in words'. However, this can obviously lead to problems of interpretation

Valid consent

- For a consent to be valid it must be made voluntarily by an informed competent patient

Competence or capacity

- The criteria of capacity that must be satisfied before the law is based on understanding rather than status (i.e. age or mental capacity). A minor's capacity to understand is thus more important than their age when allowing girls under the age of 16 to seek advice on contraception without parental consent and it is reiterated in Part IV of the Mental Health Act (1983) which recognizes that a person suffering from 'mental disorder' may consent to or refuse treatment if 'the patient is capable of doing so'. 'Every adult is presumed to have capacity, but it is a presumption that can be rebutted.'

Informed

- Adequate information must be given to allow the patient to make a balanced viewed of the benefits and faults of the treatment options

Voluntariness

- Consent should not be forced, coerced, manipulated and any consent obtained in this manner of undue influence may be deemed invalid

BATTERY AND NEGLIGENCE

- A doctor who acts without obtaining a patient's consent or ignores their refusal may be exposed in law to the civil charge of tort of battery, or tort of negligence, and in theory the criminal charge of battery

Battery

- The word battery may conjure up images of violence but in fact the term has a wider definition and includes *'being touched without consent'*. Actual physical harm does not have to be proved as harm in this context is seen as symbolic and can be committed even if the doctor acts in the patient's best interest. In England, few patients have successfully sued a doctor for battery unless no consent had been obtained in any form or they are 'involving deliberate, hostile acts.'

Negligence

- Guidelines for the legal duty for a doctor to inform patients about aspects of their treatment were first formed by the House of Lords when it was stated that 'The true test for establishing negligence in diagnosis or treatment on the part of the doctor is whether he has been proved to be guilty of such failure as no doctor of ordinary skill would be guilty of if acting with ordinary care'. In general 'A doctor is not negligent if he acts in accordance with a practice accepted at the time by a responsible body of medical opinion even though other doctors may follow a different practice. The law imposes a duty of care from the doctor to the patient but the standard of care is a matter of medical opinion 'decided primarily on the basis of expert medical evidence.'

Consent by others

- A patient normally makes the decision whether to consent to surgery but in some situations this is not possible or consent is refused. Consent can occasionally be authorized from other sources. In general age and competence (having capacity) provide the criteria as to whether this consent can be legally given by another.

The competent adult

- No adult can give consent for surgery other than the patient, and a competent adult has the right to withhold consent even if this will lead to death. This refusal does not amount to suicide in law as the patient is not directly causing his own death. Any treatment of a competent patient without consent is only lawful if covered by statute such as The Mental Health Act (1983) that allows medical treatment for the mental disorder (see below). The only exception to this is in emergencies where the patient is temporarily incompetent (i.e.

their consent cannot be obtained). To proceed without consent in this situation, the emergency intervention must be both necessary and cannot be reasonably delayed. It still can only be performed if no anticipatory refusal has been issued (i.e. such as refusal of blood products if the patient is a Jehovah's witness). Once such a refusal has been made either orally or in writing no necessity can justify intervention against it without consent

The competent child

- A refusal to consent by a competent child can be countermanded by those with 'parental responsibility'. A competent child may therefore give consent but may not withhold it in the same way

The incompetent adult

- In a similar manner to a competent adult no one can act as a true proxy for an incompetent adult. No spouse, relative or guardian of the incompetent adult has the authority to authorize consent. In specific cases to circumvent this problem The House of Lords has occasionally made the treating doctor a quasi-proxy (after taking advice from a body of medical opinion) who is directed to 'act in the best interests of the patient'. The courts give necessity rather than emergency as reason for this justification

The incompetent child

- If a child does not have the capacity to provide consent a proxy may do so. Proxy are expected to act in the best interests of the child and can include:
  - a parent who has 'parental responsibility' in respect of a child
  - a local authority that has acquired parental responsibility

In such a case the child's parents retain 'parental responsibility' and the power of consent. A local authority can only usurp this power by restricting their powers as parents. The court can act as proxy in wardship, under inherent jurisdiction or under court orders. In this way it can 'review' a parents decision (e.g. the refusal of a life giving blood transfusion for a child of a Jehovah's witness.)

Wardship

- If the child is a ward of court 'the court is entitled and bound in appropriate cases to make decisions in the interests of the child which override the rights of its parents'. Wardship may not be invoked by the local authority or while a child is in care but may be made by other interested parties (i.e. a health authority) and may end when a child ceases to be a minor. This is a major step to take as when evoked 'no important step in the life of that child, can be taken without the consent of court'.

Inherent jurisdiction

- Inherent jurisdiction is therefore more commonly used in medical law cases. The court does not take all the decisions relating to the child's life but only in certain issues, e.g. medical care. It can be invoked in an emergency and by a local authority even whilst the child is in care

Court orders

- The court also has the power to make specific orders and prohibited step orders. A prohibited step order means that no step (specified in the order) could be taken by any person including the parent without the consent of the court. A specific issue order gives directions to determine a specific question in connection with any aspect of parental responsibility for a child. These orders cannot be made if a child is in care or in an emergency and are rarely made if the child is 16 years old. They do not represent a true order as they only authorize a local authority to authorize and supervise a policy. As with all treatment the final decision and duty of care still rests with the doctor in charge of the case

ETHICS[34]

The main principles can be summarized as:

- To do no harm
- Not to assist suicide or administer euthanasia
- Not to procure abortion
- To refer patients for specialist treatment
- Not to abuse professional relationships, especially for sexual motives
- To keep the patient's confidences

DECLARATIONS

- The Declaration of Geneva attempts to govern the whole scope of medical practice. Other Declarations have been adopted which deal with more specific issues, e.g. The Declaration of Oslo (1970) deals with the question of abortion and codes of conduct based not on absolute values but on consensus opinion, which may change with time. The International Code of Medical Ethics states 'I will maintain the utmost respect for human life from the time of conception'. The Declaration of Helsinki (revised in 1975) sets out the conventions governing clinical research and human experimentation. Among its most important propositions is the need for a clearly formulated protocol describing the proposed research to be agreed by an independent committee. The Declaration of Tokyo (1975) deals with the doctor's approach to torture and other cruel, in-human or degrading treatment or punishment in relation to detention and imprisonment. 'The doctor shall in all circumstances be bound to alleviate the distress of his fellow men, and no motive whether personal, collective or political shall prevail against this higher purpose.'

CRITERIA FOR A SURGEON[9]

- Interpersonal skills
- Communication skills
- Responsibility and leadership skills
- Evaluate and analytical skills
- Broad and balanced perspective
- Decision making skills
- Personal organizational skills
- Stress tolerance
- Self motivation
- Political awareness
- Self insight and integrity
- Basic skills and abilities
- Basic academic ability
- Technical competence (including manual dexterity, good eye–hand coordination, spatial skills and a capacity for focused and sustained attention)

Key	Books	Authors/editors	Publishers
1.	The Oxford Textbook of Medicine	Weatherall	Oxford University Press
2.	Essential Urology	Bullock, Sibley and Whittaker	Churchill Livingstone
3.	Surgery	Jarell and Carabesi	Williams & Wilkins
4.	Clinical Manual of Urology	Hanno and Wein	McGraw Hill
5.	Essential Surgical Practice	Cuscheri, Giles and Moossa	Butterworth-Heinemann
6.	The New Airds Companion in Surgical Studies	Burnand and Young	Churchill Livingstone
7.	Manual clinical Oncology UICC	Love	Springer
8.	Bailey and Love's Short Practice of Surgery	Mann, Russell and Williams	Chapman & Hall
9.	Oxford Textbook of Surgery	Morris and Malt	Oxford University Press
10.	Churchill's Pocketbook of Surgery	Raftery	Churchill Livingstone
11.	The RCS Step Course	RCS	RCS
12.	An Introduction to the Signs and Symptoms of Surgical Disease	Browse	Arnold
13.	Clinical Medicine	Kumar and Clark	Ballière Tindall
14.	Clinical Surgery in General	Kirk, Mansfield and Cochrane	Churchill Livingstone
15.	Principles of Operative Surgery	Poston	Churchill Livingstone
16.	Lectures Notes Clinical Surgery	Ellis and Calne	Blackwell
17.	Surgical Secrets	Harken and Moore	Mosby
18.	Surgery (periodical)		Lumley Medicine International
19.	The Fellowship Short Answer Paper	Smiddy	Blackwell
20.	Apley's System of Orthopaedics and Fractures	Apley and Solomon	Butterworth-Heinemann
21.	Aids to Postgraduate Surgery	Watkins, Meirion and Thomas	Churchill Livingstone
22.	Essential Orthopaedics	Dandy	Churchill Livingstone
23.	Lecture Notes in Orthopaedics	Duckworth	Blackwell
24.	Practical Fracture Treatment	McCrae	Churchill Livingstone
25.	Essential Surgery	Burkitt, Quick and Gatt	Churchill Livingstone
26.	Pathology for the Primary FRCS	Gardner and Tweedle	Arnold
27.	Key Topics in Orthopaedics	Nugent, Ivory and Ross	BIOS
28.	Key Topics in Surgery	Lattimer, Wilson and Lagattolla	BIOS
29.	Current Surgical Diagnosis and Treatment	Way	Lange
30.	ATLS Student Manual		RCS
31.	Key Topics in Trauma	Greaves, Porter and Burke	BIOS
32.	Postgraduate Surgery	Al Fallouji and McBrien	Butterworth-Heinemann
33.	ABC of Colorectal Disease	Jones and Irving	British Medical Journal
34.	Fundamentals of Surgical Practice	Aljafri and Kingsnorth	Greenwich Medical Media
35.	LN Anaesthesia	Lunn	Blackwell

INDEX

U